Praise
The Future of

T0017300

"*The Future of Alzheimer's* by Sharon Ricardi offers a trove of valuable insights from experts to a question that stumps every family when a loved one is handed a diagnosis. What's next?"

—MERYL COMER,
  co-founder of UsAgainstAlzheimer's and
  author of *Slow Dancing with a Stranger*

"*The Future of Alzheimer's* is, I believe, an essential read for every family with a loved one experiencing Alzheimer's! Sharon Ricardi has collected in one place essential advice from experts and patients that truly does offer insight, inspiration, and hope. When someone is newly diagnosed with Alzheimer's or worries that they may have it, this book offers a compassionate, informed basis through which to measure expectations for the future."

—HONORABLE RICHARD T. MOORE,
  former Massachusetts State Senator and
  Chair of the Legislature's Committee on
  Health Care Financing

"This is an excellent collection of useful information from a nice variety of contributors. People with a parent newly diagnosed rarely have any idea what to do or whom to consult. This material really provides good direction for them."

—BEN PEARCE,
President of Senior Living Consulting, LLC and author of *Senior Living Communities*

the future
of alzheimer's

finding inspiration & hope
through expert insight

sharon ricardi

Hatherleigh Press is committed to preserving
and protecting the natural resources of the earth.
Environmentally responsible and sustainable practices
are embraced within the company's mission statement.

Visit us at www.hatherleighpress.com.

The Future of Alzheimer's

Library of Congress Cataloging-in-Publication Data
is available.
ISBN: 978-1-57826-986-0

COVER AND INTERIOR DESIGN BY CAROLYN KASPER

Printed in the United States
10 9 8 7 6 5 4 3 2

"For millions of Americans, the heartbreak of watching a loved one struggle with Alzheimer's disease is a pain they know all too well. Alzheimer's disease burdens an increasing number of our Nation's elders and their families, and it is essential that we confront the challenge it poses to our public health."

—PRESIDENT BARACK OBAMA

Contents

Introduction:
Why This Book, Why Now?

W HY THIS BOOK? PERHAPS the better question is, "Why this book *now?*"

I have been working in senior care for over 30 years—currently in senior living and previously in home care, always with a specialty in Alzheimer's disease. Alzheimer's, which 30 years ago was a bit of an unusual diagnosis, imperfectly understood, is now well-discussed and researched, yet still imperfectly understood despite having an enormous impact on successful aging world-wide. Indeed, it has now reached epidemic levels for millions of seniors and consumes a tremendous amount of time, money, and attention . . . including my own.

First described in 1906 by Dr. Alois Alzheimer, Alzheimer's disease is the most common form of dementia, accounting for 60–80 percent of cases. It is characterized by problems with memory, thinking and behavior. Onset is most common in individuals aged 65 and over, although people in their 40's and 50's can develop what is classed as early-onset Alzheimer's.

Alzheimer's is a progressive disease, meaning memory loss is mild in the beginning, but it worsens over time to the extent that individuals are unable to have conversations or respond to their environment. There are treatments that have been approved by the US Food and Drug Administration (FDA) for Alzheimer's. For example, cholinesterase inhibitors and memantine can help treat memory and thinking problems. But these drugs just help manage the symptoms; there is currently no cure for the disease. Alzheimer's prevalence in the US makes it the sixth leading cause of death, killing more than half a million people, mainly seniors, every year. To put this in perspective, Alzheimer's disease currently kills more people each year than prostate cancer and breast cancer combined.

The Alzheimer's Association tells us:

- Every year the world sees nearly 10 million new cases.
- The World Health Organization states that more than 55 million people have dementia worldwide, over 60% of whom live in low-and middle-income countries.
- In 2019, dementia cost economies globally 1.3 trillion US dollars.
- An estimated 6.7 million Americans aged 65 and older are living with Alzheimer's dementia in 2023. Eighty percent are aged 75 or older.
- One in 9 people aged 65 and older (10.7% percent) has Alzheimer's dementia.
- Almost two-thirds of Americans with Alzheimer's are women.
- Older African Americans are about twice as likely to have Alzheimer's or other dementias as older whites.
- Hispanics are about one and one-half times as likely to have Alzheimer's or other dementias as older whites.

As the number of older Americans grows rapidly, so too will the number of new and existing cases of Alzheimer's. By 2050, the number of people aged 65 and older with Alzheimer's dementia may grow to a projected 13.8 million, barring the development of medical breakthroughs to prevent, slow or cure Alzheimer's disease. Even now, before this tsunami of age and disease coalesce, it is sobering to realize that in the U.S. alone, a person is diagnosed with Alzheimer's every 67 seconds.

As we now know from research into the subject, Latinos and African Americans are at disproportionately greater risk of developing Alzheimer's and other dementias. The exact reasons for these differences are not fully understood, but researchers believe that their higher rates of vascular disease put them at higher risk for dementia as well. As a society, we will also need to deal with the implications of more seniors without adequate access to care.

The top ten countries that are most affected by Alzheimer's include (in the order of highest rate): **Finland, United States, Canada, Iceland, Sweden, Switzerland, Norway, Denmark, Netherlands, and**

Belgium. Those with the lowest rates include **India, Cambodia, Georgia, and Singapore.**

Studies have shown that the majority of early onset Alzheimer's cases are inherited-a form of the condition known as familial Alzheimer's disease (FAD). FAD can be caused by one of an array of gene mutations found on chromosomes 21, 14, and 1. Researchers have found that these gene mutations can lead to the development of abnormal proteins in the brain. For example, mutations on chromosome 21 can cause formation of abnormal amyloid precursor protein (APP). Most research is focused on non-FAD Alzheimer's cases, because they represent by far the greatest number of affected seniors.

Many researchers, such as Heather Snyder, PhD, the vice-president of Medical and Scientific Relations at the Alzheimer's Association, are now acknowledging the deep roots of the disease that pre-date symptoms. In her words, "Evidence suggests that the process of Alzheimer's disease begins more than a decade before clinical symptoms appear, suggesting we may need to intervene earlier to have a major impact on the course of the disease, particularly when using therapies designed to prevent the development of abnormal protein structures—plaques and tangles—that are abundant in the brains of people with Alzheimer's."

On a personal note, my early training in preparation for my role in home care taught us to "reorient the poor delusional patient to time and place." Which we did, over and over . . . for a while, at least. Then, many of us, myself included, realized how fruitless and indeed cruel it was to continually remind someone who clearly was unable to remember our carefully reasoned message of how their mother, for example, could not possibly still be alive as that would make her 130 years old! So, slowly, the rules were rewritten to be more knowledgeable and compassionate.

Finally, in the 1990s real training became available for the disease, much of it sponsored by the local Alzheimer's Associations. My own training was through the Massachusetts Alzheimer's Association, specifically by the brilliant Joanne Koenig Coste (author of the internationally acclaimed book "*Speaking Alzheimer's*") and Dr. Paul Raia, former Vice President of the Massachusetts Alzheimer's

Association, who continues to advocate for those with the disease. While well-known now, at the time their groundbreaking "habilitation" approach opened many eyes to new ways to care for those on the long journey. Then many in the field turned their attention to treatment, indeed, for quite a while it was believed that a good pharmacological treatment would be easily found.

At first, we in the senior care field eagerly grasped at anything that offered the promise of staving off the worst affects for months or even years. One can understand the desire to find a suitable treatment, as scientists estimate that if an effective treatment is not found soon, by 2050 someone in the United States will develop the disease every 33 seconds, twice the current rate.

This drug-based approach, most significantly the early drug Donepezil (sold under the brand name Aricept) had some success, but ultimately proved elusive and somewhat disappointing because when the therapy was stopped the typical recipient quickly progressed to where they would have been without the drugs. In addition, there are many potential side effects and a need for close medical monitoring. The typical downward outcome when the drug is stopped was often crushing for families.

The Food and Drug Administration (FDA) has approved different types of drugs specifically to treat symptoms of Alzheimer's disease. According to the FDA, these drugs are approved for specific stages of Alzheimer's. These stages—mild, moderate, and severe—are based on scores on tests that assess memory, awareness of time and place, and thinking and reasoning.

One way Alzheimer's disease harms the brain is by decreasing levels of a chemical messenger (acetylcholine) that's important for alertness, memory, thought and judgment. Cholinesterase (ko-lin-ES-tur-ays) inhibitors boost the amount of acetylcholine available to nerve cells by preventing its breakdown in the brain.

Cholinesterase inhibitors can't reverse Alzheimer's disease or stop the destruction of nerve cells. These medications eventually lose effectiveness because dwindling brain cells produce less acetylcholine as the disease progresses.

Three cholinesterase inhibitors that are FDA approved and commonly prescribed are:

- **Donepezil (Aricept)** is approved to treat all stages of the disease. It's taken once a day as a pill.
- **Galantamine (Razadyne)** is approved to treat mild to moderate Alzheimer's. It's taken as a pill once a day or as an extended-release capsule twice a day.
- **Rivastigmine (Exelon)** is approved for mild to moderate Alzheimer's disease. It's taken as a pill. A skin patch is available that can also be used to treat severe Alzheimer's disease.

For those in the later stages, Memantine (Namenda) is approved by the FDA for treatment of moderate to severe Alzheimer's disease. It works by regulating the activity of glutamate, a messenger chemical widely involved in brain functions—including learning and memory.

The FDA has also approved a combination of donepezil and memantine (Namzaric), which is taken as a capsule.

After nearly twenty years of false starts and little progress in the search for effective treatments, let alone a cure, in 2021 the first of what are now three promising treatments surfaced.

The much-heralded and newly approved drug for early stage Alzheimer's is Aducanumab. It is an amyloid beta-directed monoclonal antibody. This infusion therapy is approved only for patients with mild cognitive impairment and mild dementia due to Alzheimer's disease. Approval was given for Aduhelm understanding that FDA approval was premature, but with the desire to give some relief to those suffering with the disease. As the FDA stated, it can be prescribed while another study is being conducted because the "need for treatments is urgent." In addition, Biogen, the maker of Aduhelm, cut in half the amount they planned to charge for this treatment, which consists of every other week infusions, from $56,400 to $28,200 per year.

Following closely on the heels of Aduhelm was lacanemab, to be sold as Leqembi. This too received accelerated FDA approval and shows about a 30% slowing of the effects of Alzheimer's. It also has been shown in clinical trials to have less side effects that Aduhelm. Finally, at the time of this writing, the most recent drug, donanemab, which is also a monoclonal antibody, is also given via infusions, is in the early stages of trials. It is proving to be similarly effective, with similar potential side effects, namely brain bleeds. It is the third new Alzheimer's drug expected to be approved by the Food and Drug Administration.

At long last, the field is beginning to show progress in the fight to slow the disease. While this is exciting news, these drugs work best for those in the earliest stages of Alzheimer's, and other therapies will need to be developed to help those with advanced disease. And none of them are able to reverse or repair existing damage to the brain.

While this is likely "just the opening chapter in a new era of molecular therapies for Alzheimer's disease and related neurodegenerative disorders," as Gil Rabinovici, MD, director of the UCSF Alzheimer's Disease Research Center, wrote in a July 17, 2023, JAMA editorial, it is, undoubtedly, a hopeful start.

Importantly, The Centers for Medicare and Medicaid Services (CMS) recently announced that, consistent with CMS' National Coverage Determination document issued on April 7, 2022, Medicare will now cover and pay for drugs in the class of monoclonal antibodies directed against amyloid for the treatment of Alzheimer's disease with traditional FDA approval. To obtain coverage, the provider participates in a data submission effort, commonly referred to as a registry, to further evaluate whether the drug is reasonable and necessary in the Medicare population. It is hard to overstate how important this decision is relative to the need for health equity in the United States.

Over and over again, I hear how research is providing growing evidence that brain health is even more closely linked to heart and blood vessel health. And just like the treatments for heart health, lifestyle choices matter. Alzheimer's is indeed proving to be a complex and formidable foe, and future treatments may be more of a cocktail of different medications similar to the successful treatment developed for HIV-AIDS that has allowed those with AIDS to live with what was only recently considered a death sentence. While hope for a cure or more successful treatment continues, we in the caregiving field still focus on learning how to best care for those already dealing with the disease.

The best teachers, it should be no surprise, turned out to be the seniors who actually had Alzheimer's. Listening to them, being in the moment with them, and paying attention to their nonverbal "language" taught us all so much. While training is so important, if I had to remind people of one thing, it is that every single person with Alzheimer's is on their own journey, unique to them, so prepare for the fact that what you learned from observing one person, what you read and heard will almost certainly be at least slightly different with your own loved one. And why not? We are all so different, and we must be treated that way.

One resident of the first assisted living community I oversaw, a sweet woman named Hazel from a prominent Boston family, had initially been living in the traditional assisted living side of the community. She always loved it when we went to the Boston Ballet, knew every symphony, and was on all the prominent social committees. When a few years later she needed to transition to our memory care wing due to her advancing Alzheimer's putting her at risk of wandering, I was concerned that she would find the activities there, which are simpler, a little on the childish side. I went to see her one day after a group of memory care residents had just returned from an outing with baby barnyard animals. Her face was wreathed in smiles, and I said "Hazel, you look like you really enjoyed your trip today." It was as if she read my mind. She grasped my hand, leaned in, and said: "My dear, everything does not have to be Mozart to make me happy!"

For the last twenty years, my roles have included regional oversight of dementia units in assisted living, and then corporate director of memory care. In those roles, I have tried to understand how a thoughtfully therapeutic environment can best make life not just bearable, but often enjoyable for seniors dealing with this diagnosis. That direction has been rewarding, as the more we learn, the more we can redesign the physical environment and more finely tune our associate training. And in a perfect feedback loop, the more we see results, the more we are able to guide the way.

People—be it family, friends, or care staff— approach the resident in every interaction. We have looked at enhancing the dining experience, the lighting, the overall design flow, and the rhythm of the day, ensuring that it allows for sufficient sleep and exercise. Never forgotten is the need to provide joyful, appropriate entertainment and purpose filled activities that allow the senior to be happy in the moment. We have come so far in making the best of a fraught situation. But still, we come to love our residents like family, and so we yearn for a cure.

I have worked with some wonderful colleagues in the field, each of whom has added to my knowledge and understanding of Alzheimer's. I have often shared their thoughts with others I speak with, as well as family and friends or even strangers that I meet who are on the journey. (Even as I write this I am on a cruise from England to the Canary Islands and just this morning, over breakfast, a fellow cruiser asked what I did and then, as her husband drank a second cup of coffee, she tearfully told me her mother's story and begged for advice on how to handle the heart-break of her mother not recognizing her when she visited her care home in Sussex.) The heartbreak, I hear is deeply personal and real, and I always strive to imbue hope in any of my comments. They go to their doctors for medical advice, but still need reassurance. One particular quote that I have loved for years and I shared with her was:

> *My happiness grows in direct proportion to*
> *my acceptance, and in inverse proportion to*
> *my expectations.*
> —MICHAEL J. FOX

This quote by the beloved actor Michael J. Fox, who suffers from but does not give in to Parkinson's, affirms two things: happiness can exist again, but also acceptance cannot be cheated. Learning, accepting, and finding joy in the small successes has worked in my life, and I recommend it to others. Accepting what is happening to your loved one is the first step to directing your attention towards cherishing what has not changed and finding moments to be cherished in the small moments. I also always ask others in the field how they best help families accept what is happening—what words have the most impact, what reassurances are true yet comforting.

Recently it was suggested that I write down the best of the insights that I have gleaned. At first, I resisted; I do, as my family well knows, have a long-neglected fictional manuscript languishing on my laptop. The idea percolated, however. I thought, 'Would I like to read a book like this? Would I give it to someone caring for a loved one with an Alzheimer's diagnosis, or working in this field? Could these words make a difference to someone?'

A clear "yes" finally spurred me to collect my notes, reach out to more experts and collect their thoughts on the two questions I always want insight on:

1. **In the here and now, what advice can we offer for those who cannot wait for a cure?**
2. **Do you think there will be a cure, and if so, when?**

As I was in the early stages of writing this book, the COVID-19 pandemic took hold. It distracted and delayed me from completion, as I am still very active in the healthcare consulting field and our clients needed help in dealing with all the implications and devastation of so many lives lost. But as I was close to finishing the book, the news broke that in a mere (relatively speaking) nine months a COVID-19 vaccine was researched, developed, and tested and ready for approval and distribution. In nine months! It made me wonder what could happen if we gave that much global time, research money, and attention to finding a cure or successful treatment for Alzheimer's.

As you will read, many of the quotes contained in this book are from leaders in the Alzheimer's research field, working diligently on understanding the disease with the goal of finding a cure, while others are caring and experienced dementia professionals dealing with the challenges of the here and now. Others are caregivers who rose to the challenge. Many have written books on the subject that I found useful, and others run companies that faithfully and often heroically deal with the here and now of care. There are also quotes from important people in my life who represent those that have experienced this illness on a personal level.

My office bookshelves are full of books on this topic, many informative and perspective-changing, many almost unbearably intimate and heartbreaking, most unfailingly proving the resiliency of our fellow human beings. I have collected a selection in the references section of this book that you may want to read, when you are ready.

Come on this journey with me and look inside the hearts and minds of those who are dedicated to making Alzheimer's less of the devastating diagnosis it is now.

> *It's now known that the brain can form new axons and dendrites up to the last years of life, which gives us tremendous hope for preventing senility, for example, and preserving our mental capacity indefinitely.*
>
> **—RUDOLPH E. TANZI**

Note: *The medical profession is slowly transitioning the name for this disease from Alzheimer's Disease to Alzheimer Disease, as they did with transitioning Down's Syndrome to Down Syndrome. I have chosen to retain the historical form in this book to not cause confusion.*

You may also note the many local sources of quotes. I now live in Plymouth MA, and prior to that in Sandwich and Cotuit MA, all towns defined by the embrace of the sea that surrounds us on and just off Cape Cod. The Alzheimer's community of the Cape and Islands is a tight knit community and very supportive of each other, hence there are many connections made. In addition, Boston turns out to be one of the leading hot beds of Alzheimer's research in the world.

Carpe Diem

John Zeisel PhD, Hon. D. Sc.

I am pleased to count Dr. Zeisel among the many influences in my education on the puzzle that is understanding and assisting those with Alzheimer's. Being a fellow Massachusetts resident, I had the opportunity to discuss with him the role the assisted living industry plays in this field and observe first-hand the influence he has had in changing the perception of caregivers towards this particular challenge experienced by far too many of the elderly.

Dr. Zeisel is a national and global leader in the compassionate ethical care of elders living in Assisted Living settings with an emphasis on those living with Alzheimer's and other dementias. He is the founder of both Hearthstone, a Massachusetts firm that manages memory care communities, and the I'm Still Here® Foundation, a not-for-profit organization that supports the development of dementia-specific nonpharmacologic treatment interventions.

Dr. Zeisel received a Ph.D. in Sociology from Columbia University, he was awarded a Fellowship at the National Institute for Advanced Studies near The Hague in the Netherlands. He served on the Board of Directors of Abe's Garden, the Patient Care and Family Support Committee of the Massachusetts Alzheimer's Association, and the International Advisory Board of the Academy for Health and Design and was a founding member of the Board of Directors of the Academy for Neuroscience in Architecture. His publications include, I'm Still Here: A New Approach to Dementia Care, *and* Inquiry by Design: Environment/Behavior/Neuroscience for Architects, Interiors, Landscape and Planning *and numerous professional journal articles.*

What advice would you give to the loved ones of someone newly diagnosed?

You probably feel like a tree just fell on you and that there is no escape. You feel like the only alternative is a downward spiral of despair from now on for the rest of your life. It doesn't have to be that way—you can make a difference in your and your loved one's life by how you approach living with dementia—how you embrace life. You have years in front of you of travel, awareness, entertainment, opinions, family and friends, sports events, and broadcasts, and so much more. And it is up to you to grab the day: *Carpe diem*.

First grieve that you and the person you love will be living with a chronic condition there is no way out of. But don't let that grief dominate you and the way you see and act in the world. *Hope* lies in knowing that you are still you, no matter what. *Hope* lies in knowing that *You Can Make a Difference* (YCMAD) in the quality of your life together—the way you live, speak to each other, the way you enjoy life—in so many ways. *Carpe diem*.

> **Hope lies in knowing that you are still you, no matter what.**

Do you think there will be a cure? And if so, when?

It is unlikely that a 'cure' for Alzheimer's will be developed in the foreseeable future because it is a condition whose main correlate is old age. There will be no 'cure' for old age, and there shouldn't be because old age is not an illness, it is a phase of life. Researchers around the globe are learning more about the brain every day, and with that knowledge comes the hope that one day we will live in a world where Alzheimer's does not exist.

> **There will be no 'cure' for old age, and there shouldn't be because old age is not an illness, it is a phase of life.**

Until that time, as with other conditions we live with and at whatever age, the best thing to do for people with dementia is deliver programs and approaches that reduce apparent symptoms and provide the highest quality of life. In dementia, this means first recognizing that the person is *still here*; then organizing the physical environment, personal supports, and the social surroundings—the person's *Eco psychosocial* environment—to help them be the full person they have been, they are, and they will always be.

To love a person is to learn the song in their heart and sing it to them when they have forgotten.
—ANNE GARBORG

Do Not Define the Person By the Disease

Peter Reed, PhD

I have learned much by reading the many papers and book chapters written by Dr. Peter Reed. He is the Director of the Sanford Center for Aging and Professor of Community Health Sciences at the University of Nevada, Reno. He has over 20 years of experience in the field of aging that bridges research, practice, policy, and organizational leadership.

Dr. Reed has a Ph.D. and MPH in Health Behavior and Health Education from the School of Public Health at the University of North Carolina at Chapel Hill, where he was a National Institute on Aging Pre-Doctoral Fellow in the Carolina Program on Healthcare and Aging Research.

He served as Chief Executive Officer of the Pioneer Network, President and CEO of the Center for Health Improvement and Senior Director of Programs for the

Alzheimer's Association National Office, where he led the Association's Program Division in developing and delivering a wide range of care and support programs for people living with Alzheimer's nationwide.

A frequent author and public speaker, Dr. Reed has published over 50 papers, monographs, and book chapters in peer-reviewed and industry publications. His take on the disease is, however, decidedly humanistic and hopeful.

What advice would you give to the loved ones of someone newly diagnosed?

I would help them to understand that a significant part of diminished quality of life related to dementia is the result of stigma and society's reaction to the disease, above and beyond the impact of the disease itself. The response to a diagnosis can be as damaging as the disease. I would help them understand that a person living with dementia should not be defined by the disease experience, but rather can and should remain an active, engaged member of their family and community. There will be a need for additional support to adapt and accommodate some dementia-related changes, but that support should be offered in a way that is mindful of the person's interests and preferences and should achieve a balance between personal autonomy and physical safety to ensure a person's basic human rights are preserved.

Do not make assumptions about what a person living with dementia cannot or should not do, as focusing on limitations will only serve to limit the person. Instead, remain focused on retained abilities and ensuring that the person's everyday life is not medicalized in ways that deprive them of their personhood. The dominant narrative in the field of Alzheimer's disease is one of tragedy that shapes a negative characterization of people living with the disease and directly neglects a human-centered, supportive approach grounded in maintaining dignity, respect and opportunities for continued growth and joy. Do not define the person by the disease.

" I would help them understand that a person living with dementia should not be defined by the disease experience, but rather can and should remain an active, engaged member of their family and community. "

Do you believe there will be a cure? And if so, when?

I am not a biomedical researcher, so I am not qualified to comment on the specifics of the research currently underway for a disease-modifying drug. However, I can say that dementia is a multifactorial condition rooted in genetic, environmental, social, and behavioral factors. The idea that a 'cure' is going to address these numerous factors seems unlikely. In my view, it is a misdirection to set a goal of a world without dementia but would rather be more appropriate to focus on how, with or without effective treatments, we can create a world that supports people with varying cognitive abilities in living well. Further, even if a 'cure' were developed, the health inequity and disparities created by social determinants of health that are a central feature of the capitalist medical system in the US would prevent access to millions of people who could benefit from the treatment. The impact of a new treatment cannot be considered outside the context of barriers to accessing care for large segments of the population.

> ❝ In my view, it is a misdirection to set a goal of a world without dementia but would rather be more appropriate to focus on how, with or without effective treatments, we can create a world that supports people with varying cognitive abilities in living well. ❞

I am seeking, I am not lost.
I am forgetful, I am not gone.

—JOANNE KOENIG COSTE

Education, Education, Education.

Rachael Wonderlin

Rachael Wonderlin is a busy author, blogger, and consultant in the field of Alzheimer's and related dementia. Rachael has a master's degree in Gerontology and works as a dementia care consultant through her own company, Dementia by Day. Author of four books on Alzheimer's, Rachael's most popular book, When Someone You Know Is Living in a Dementia Care Community, *is one I highly recommend. I enjoyed conversing with Rachael about her take on how the understanding of how to interact with those with Alzheimer's has changed over the years.*

A passage in her book that I particularly liked is "You may find it challenging to figure out which stage your friend or family member is in however, because two people with Alzheimer's Disease can experience the disease very differently. For example, one 80-year-old woman with Alzheimer's may stay in an advanced stage of dementia for four years. Another woman of the same age may spend five months in a moderate stage before suddenly becoming more advanced in her dementia and passing away." This advice is so helpful to families who want to learn as much as they can to prepare themselves but need to be able to accept different paths taken by different people.

What advice would you give to the loved ones of someone newly diagnosed?

The number one piece of advice that I share is this: educate yourself and your loved ones about dementia. I truly believe that education—or the lack thereof—is the number one reason that people excel or fail. I don't mean a formal education, either (although I do deeply believe in formal education) but in the idea that one needs to continue to learn, seek knowledge, question what they hear, and reach out to others.

"With the right dementia education and knowledge of your choices, you can know that you're doing the right thing."

Read, listen, join a support group, go to events, journal your feelings and thoughts. All of these are crucial.

When someone finds me to ask a dementia care question, it's almost always the same one. The question is some variation of, "Am I making the right choice?" or, "Am I doing the right thing?" Families feel an immense amount of guilt and anxiety over making choices for their loved ones with cognitive impairments, and they constantly question whether or not they are "doing the right thing." With the right dementia education and knowledge of your choices, you can know that you're doing the right thing.

A person who has a diagnosis often feels anxious and isolated. They're afraid that people won't understand, or they can see people pulling away from them because the individuals don't know what to do. Education, education, education.

Don't forget that your thoughts and feelings are important. I highly recommend, in the very least, writing a couple sentences down each day about how you are doing.

Do you think there will be a cure? And if so, when?

This is a complicated question, because there are over 100 different causes of cognitive loss. In fact, researchers fairly recently discovered another cause that they'd previously mistaken with Alzheimer's disease: LATE, or limbic-predominant age-related TDP-43 encephalopathy.

I think that there will be, in the very least, ways to slow or stop the effects of certain dementias. Even a decade ago, most everyone felt pretty hopeless about a cure for HIV. Today, in the US, many people are able to live with HIV—we haven't completely eradicated the health crisis surrounding HIV and AIDS, but we've made massive steps in that direction.

I believe we're going to see similar progress with many causes of dementia.

> *" I think that there will be, in the very least, ways to slow or stop the effects of certain dementias. "*

I know of no single formula for success. But over the years I have observed that some attributes of leadership are universal and are often about finding ways of encouraging people to combine their efforts, their talents, their insights, their enthusiasm and their inspiration to work together.

—HER MAJESTY QUEEN
ELIZABETH II

Reduce Your Risk

Lauren Aguirre

Lauren is the author of an amazing new book called The Memory Thief. *This book is a finalist for the 2022 Pen/E.O. Wilson Literary Science Writing Award. I received it as a Christmas gift in December 2021, and read it voraciously, as it reads like a thriller but is filled with new discoveries about how the memory works.*

She is an award-winning science journalist who has produced documentaries, short-form video series, podcasts, interactive games, and blogs for the PBS series NOVA. *While she has covered everything from asteroids to human origins to art restoration, it turns out she, like me, is particularly fascinated by the brain.*

What advice would you give to the loved ones of someone newly diagnosed?

If you have a picture in your mind of what it's like to have Alzheimer's, try your best to put it aside. Every person's trajectory is different. And even though current treatments at best reduce symptoms for a period of time, it is not too late to take steps to help you, or your family manage the decline in ways that can offer many more years of a meaningful life.

> *Every person's trajectory is different.*

Do you think there will be a cure? And if so, when?

Based on the research I did for my book, it seems unlikely there will be a cure, but every expert I spoke with was optimistic that treatments to stave off decline are on the horizon. The timeline differed—three years, five years, ten years—but for a whole host of reasons, researchers and patients finally have reasons to hope after decades of failed and disappointing clinical trials.

For starters, the pipeline of possible treatments is expanding. Techniques for screening thousands of compounds in a petri dish can quickly identify ones that make sense to test in mice. And although mice don't get Alzheimer's, the genetically engineered animals that researchers now use to test treatments come much closer to capturing the complexity of the human disease. This level of sophistication makes it more likely that results in mice will translate into people.

As for human clinical trials, better diagnostic tools make it possible to enroll people in the early stages when interventions are more likely to succeed. New tools also ensure that the people enrolled in the trial actually have Alzheimer's. In the past, in some trials, as many as a third of participants did not.

As risk factors and the progression of the disease are better understood, "curing" Alzheimer's could be a matter of prevention.

Perhaps most importantly, researchers are no longer looking just under the spotlight. For decades, one model of the disease held sway, arguably holding back progress. But now, there is willingness, as one expert put it to me, for researchers to "take more shots on goal." Strengthening brain waves with light and sound, deep brain stimulation, taming excessive inflammation, or reducing hyperactivity in certain brain regions are just a few examples of fresh approaches. This attitude is critical because there are multiple versions of Alzheimer's. And it may be that a combination of therapies, or different treatments for different patients, will make it possible for people to live for many years with minimal symptoms.

The greatest prize, of course, would be never to develop Alzheimer's in the first place. As risk factors and the progression of the disease are better understood, "curing" Alzheimer's could be a matter of prevention—of just not getting it in the first place. Today, people at risk for heart disease take statins to ward off heart attacks. Someday, there may be similar drugs that people at risk for Alzheimer's can take. And until then, you can reduce your risk by doing everything you would do to care for your general well-being, including exercising, eating well, getting good quality sleep—and using your brain as often as possible!

> *People do not realize that Alzheimer's is not old age. It is a progressive and fatal disease and staggering amounts of people develop Alzheimer's every day.*
>
> —MELINA KANAKAREDES

Real Life is What Happens in Between the Medical Interactions

Dr. Alan Abrams

Alan Abrams has been a practicing geriatrician, physician executive and leader in geriatric education for more than 30 years. His career has been marked by leadership positions at the intersection of the provider and payer spaces. During his time as chief of geriatrics at Cambridge Health Alliance, he helped launch one of the early PACE programs in Massachusetts. He is also involved in bringing PACE (Program of All-inclusive Care for the Elderly) to Washington DC, which is where my work and his programs brought us into contact. His holistic approach to treating seniors with dementia, not to mention the depth and breadth of his practical experience in how the disease impacts health care in this country, is truly impressive. He is nationally recognized for designing model geriatric health care delivery programs for culturally diverse, low-income populations. He recently served as chief medical officer of the Pioneer Accountable Care Organization at Beth Israel Deaconess, which included Medicare shared savings risk contracts covering 70,000 lives.

Alan has also served as medical director of United-Health's Special Needs Plan for People Living in Nursing Homes, and the Cambridge Health Alliance Center for Excellence for Senior Health. He served as director of the geriatric fellowship program at Harvard Medical School and has been involved in the training of hundreds of practicing geriatricians. He is on the faculty at Harvard Medical School and continues to teach as well as speak internationally on geriatrics, education, and health care delivery for the elderly.

Dr. Abrams holds a master's in public health from the Harvard School of Public Health and an MD from the New York University School of Medicine.

What advice would you give to the loved ones of someone newly diagnosed?

What I say from my particular perspective as a geron-tologist is that what is really important for caregivers and significant others to know is that this is a chronic and progressive illness. It may seem to be quantum changes because of the way the interactions happen but that occurrence may have just happened and may not be significant. We are there to work with them.

Unlike a specialist, who feels they have got to give you something, we realize as geriatricians that we may not have the perfect solution, but we do have interventions that can help everyone involved. I also stress that they shouldn't try to do it by themselves, you have to take care of you, you have to be aware of the instinct of the medical system to want to isolate problems and try to treat beware of the hazards of hospitalization for people with Alzheimer's and of course other issues are safety awareness that needs to be a constant conversation about the increasing and changing needs for safety awareness.

Remember that being a caregiver for someone with Alzheimer's is a team sport don't think you need to do it alone it's impossible.

Nutrition is extremely important. Exercise is also very important. Try to remember they always enjoyed it and it may be more grounding for them to play a video of the 2004 Red Sox win versus taking them to a game today with all the stress that that sometimes entails. Don't be shy about repeating experiences if they like them once they'll like them again. Real life is what happens in between the medical interactions. Maximize what is enjoyable and don't worry about trying to set the human record for longevity.

Beware of polypharmacy as that can be counterproductive. At Edenbridge our KPI equals the number of days that they want to get up and enjoy the day. That should be your NorthStar as a caregiver creating enjoyable days not just focusing on the health aspects of it. Remember that being a caregiver for someone with Alzheimer's is a team sport don't think you need to do it alone, it's impossible. Get back to the exercise piece and add that he said especially mixed dementia and especially aerobic exercises. Good blood pressure management and if they have high blood pressure is a very important thing to look at.

As I continue to work with caregivers, I usually try to remind people that as people suffering with this disease, they often experience ongoing degenerative processes that imitate the newborn sensory function in reverse. Babies first respond to touch and sound then visual stimulation, then taste and smell. I always try to remind them to try to not stop touching the person with Alzheimer's that is a therapy in and of itself not just for the caregiver but for the person suffering with Alzheimer's as well.

Do you think there will be a cure? And if so, when?

Regarding this question, I think the word "cure" is the tricky part of the question. I do think that coming to your local theaters soon, there will be many ways to help people improve their neurological functioning that will fall short of an actual cure. And although we aren't sure, I would say by the year 2050 we will have research that will have made major steps toward helping reduce the neuronal loss of someone with Alzheimer's, which will increase connectivity to allow them to function more normally.

I do think that coming to your local theaters soon, there will be many ways to help people improve their neurological functioning that will fall short of an actual cure.

'There is a moral task of caregiving, and that involves just being there, being with that person and being committed. When there is nothing that can be done, we have to be able to say, 'look, I'm with you in this experience.' Right through to the end of it.'

—DR. ARTHUR KLEINMAN

A Name and Explanation

J. Cara Pendergrass, PhD

I first met Cara at her wedding to a family friend, a spectacular affair that nevertheless afforded me no time to discuss this project with her. It wasn't until a few months later that I learned of her full expertise: a Clinical Psychologist with specialty training in Neuropsychology. She is also an Associate Professor; Clinical Psychology Department; at William James College. Her affiliations include the International Neuropsychological Society, The Alzheimer's Association International Society to Advance Alzheimer's Research and Treatment, the American Psychological Association. Currently she is Vice President of Clinical Operations at Clintarra LLC.

I was particularly intrigued by her wide ranging and fascinating work as a Clinical Research Trial Consultant for Neurological and Neuropsychiatric Disorders where she is exposed to much of the latest research. Her insightful comments are included here, and provide a realistic and clinically exact understanding of the science behind my two questions.

What advice would you give to the loved ones of someone newly diagnosed?

I am frequently asked how difficult it is to confirm for an individual and their family that the individual has a diagnosis of Alzheimer's disease. I deliberately used the word 'confirm' in the previous sentence because the individual and family members have already observed that the individual is experiencing changes: changes in how the person is thinking or changes in how the person is able to do day to day activities. A diagnosis of Alzheimer's disease is never easy, but more often than not, I find that individuals and families are relieved to have a name and explanation for what is happening, even if the diagnosis is Alzheimer's disease.

Once I've answered questions about Alzheimer's disease, the current considerations of treatment and working with their neurologist (or establishing appointments with a neurologist, if needed), the most important information that I then provide is contact information for all types of support and support groups and agencies. We know that the neuropatho-physiological processes for Alzheimer's disease are complicated, but the nature of Alzheimer's disease regarding the individual's experience of progressing clinical, cognitive, and behavioral symptoms, the impact on the family, and likely future implications of caregiving also is complicated. There is extensive information as well as numerous and different types of support available that the individual and family likely does not know exists but will be crucial for both the individual and the family along all the steps going forward.

> *A diagnosis of Alzheimer's disease is never easy, but more often than not, I find that individuals and families are relieved to have a name and explanation for what is happening, even if the diagnosis is Alzheimer's disease.*

Do you think there will be a cure? And if so, when?

As simple as this statement appears, this question is rather complicated with multiple layers one must consider. Medically, the term cure implies that an individual no longer has that condition and usually refers to a restoration of health. An individual may be cured and no longer have a condition after receiving treatment. Treatment refers to a process or approach that has the purpose of leading to an improvement in health. If the treatment does result in the complete elimination of a condition, then the individual is cured of the condition.

However, a treatment may not result in the complete elimination of a condition. There are many conditions that are treatable in which a treatment intervention(s) does not cure the disease but manages the symptoms and the disease, such as diabetes and multiple sclerosis.

> " *As simple as it sounds, there are lifestyle factors which research has consistently shown to have significant protective factors for our brain functioning and reduction in risk for Alzheimer's disease.* "

Currently, there are no treatments that cure Alzheimer's. We also are very limited in the treatments available to manage the symptoms of Alzheimer's disease. Additionally, the treatments we do have available are very limited in their ability to slow the progression of Alzheimer's disease.

However, our current limitations in treatment(s) for Alzheimer's disease are not due to a lack of thousands of medical professionals all over the world continuously engaging in clinical research and working to identify and examine the efficacy of different treatment possibilities for the past few decades. As unfortunate as it is that we still do not have more efficacious treatments for Alzheimer's disease, all of these endeavors have resulted in incredible gains in our knowledge of Alzheimer's disease and, even more important, what we still do not know about Alzheimer's disease.

It can be helpful to compare the evolution to our understanding of diagnosing, classifying, and treating cancer to what has begun to unfold in our understanding of diagnosing, classifying, and ultimately treating Alzheimer's disease.

We now know that cancer includes a large group of related diseases characterized by the development of abnormal cells that divide uncontrollably. We also know that each person's cancer cells have a unique combination of genetic alterations and that certain cancer treatments are now based on the genetic testing of an individual's cancer cells to determine which treatments will work best.

For Alzheimer's disease, we now know that it is a heterogenous disorder and have begun to identify various neuropathological subtypes related to distributions of neurofibrillary tangles and associated brain atrophy. We also have learned more about other types of dementia, including Lewy Body Dementia and Frontotemporal dementia (FTD), which previously would be unintentionally misdiagnosed as Alzheimer's dementia. Better understanding the neuropathological variants of Alzheimer's disease and differential diagnosis from other dementias is crucial and essential in our ability to progress forward in identifying efficacious treatments.

Just like certain chemotherapies will work for one type of cancer but not another, our understanding of the neuropathological elements of different subtypes of Alzheimer's disease is crucial in understanding how to development treatment interventions given that one type of treatment intervention is unlikely to work for different neuropathological subtypes of Alzheimer's disease.

Research examining treatments for Alzheimer's disease over the past few decades also has identified two key distinctions in types of treatment interventions: clinical symptom treatments and disease modifying treatments. Development of treatment interventions targeting the management of the cognitive, clinical, and behavioral symptoms experienced by individuals with Alzheimer's dementia can help day-to-day functioning but may be limited in how long they are efficacious given that the underlying neuropathological processes are not impacted by the treatments.

A disease modification treatment means that the treatment intervention impacts the underlying neuropathophysiology or neuronal brain changes associated with Alzheimer's disease; however, this does not automatically translate into management and/or improvement in clinical, cognitive, or behavior symptoms of Alzheimer's disease. Currently, there are treatment interventions that have been found to impact the underlying neuropathology and help to reduce amyloid plaques in Alzheimer's disease; however, individuals still experience the progression of cognitive, clinical, and behavioral symptoms.

As frustrating as it is to find that the clinical symptoms are not impacted by the disease modification treatments, it also highlights for researchers that there are other important neuropathological factors that also are involved in and contributing to Alzheimer's disease which still must be identified and targeted for a complete, comprehensive treatment to address both the neuropathological processes and cognitive, clinical, and behavioral symptoms associated with Alzheimer's disease.

Returning to the question at hand, 'Do you believe there will be a cure, and if so, when?' The possibility of a cure some day in the future is not completely impossible as we make advances in our understanding of the neuropathophysiology of Alzheimer's disease and how these changes result in the cognitive, clinical, and behavior symptoms and through tremendous technological advances in our ability to study the brain and neuronal and neuro-pathological mechanisms.

However, we may find that Alzheimer's disease may conceptually be like high blood pressure: it is treatable without a cure, but it is also preventable. For our current day, it can be helpful to conceptualize Alzheimer's disease as a condition in which there are actions that we can take to prevent or reduce our risk of developing Alzheimer's disease. As simple as it sounds, there are lifestyle factors which research has consistently shown to have significant protective factors for our brain functioning and reduction in risk for Alzheimer's disease. Regular exercise (as little as walking 30 minutes three to four times per week) is a factor that research has consistently found to be a protective factor for cognitive functioning as we age and reduces risk in development of Alzheimer's disease. Regular sleep and healthy eating (including limited processed foods) also have been found to be protective factors.

These lifestyle factors of regular exercise, sleep, and healthy eating are the body's own mechanisms to regulate and reduce inflammatory processes and responses to various toxins, chemicals, bacteria, or tissue injury that we experience every day. Research consistently has shown that increases in inflammatory processes are a crucial factor in neuropathology of Alzheimer's Disease and progression of the disease. So, although we are limited on treatments for Alzheimer's disease currently, we do have knowledge on everyday actions that we all have available to us as neuroprotective factors: exercise, sleep, and healthy eating.

Though those with Alzheimer's might forget us, we as a society must remember them.
—SCOTT KIRSHENBAUM

Have a Community of Support Around You

Steph Jagger

Steph Jagger is the author of two books. Her first,
Unbound: A Story of Snow & Self-Discovery was
published in 2017. I read it soon after it came out, as
I am a reader of all genres and love being surprised by a
story. I also "followed her" and recently learned of her
second book, a mother-daughter story, Everything Left
to Remember, came out in April of 2022. It is a story all
too often repeated, learning your parent has Alzheimer's.
But it is what came next, a trek through the Rockies, and
her beautiful writing that lift this book out of the ordinary.
I felt she would have something meaningful to add to my
own book, as she is going through this journey right now
with her mother and "feeling the feelings" in her own way.

Outside of being an author, Steph is a sought-after
mentor, coach, speaker, and facilitator whose work lies

at the intersection of love and loss, the nature of deep remembrance, and the personal journey of re-creation.

What advice would you give to the loved ones of someone newly diagnosed?

I tell them I'm sorry and that this is awful news. I also ask them if it would be helpful for me to share three things that have helped me get through this journey. If they agree, I share the following:

1. It is easy, and will become easier, to think you are alone in this, but you are not. Reach out to other people. Talk about your experience as openly as feels good. Ask an organization like your local Alzheimer's Association Chapter for help. Do all of these things early so you have a community of support around you.

2. People will begin to ask you how the person with Alzheimer's is. This is an impossible question to answer, and I've come to believe that they're trying to ask how you are but don't really know how. I've gotten in the habit of being very honest. I tell them, "I'm not exactly sure how my mom is, but today was hard for me."

3. They will forget who you are, but you don't
   have to. Do everything you can to remind
   yourself . . . to remember who you are, as you
   move through this journey.

> *It is easy, and will become easier,
> to think you are alone in this, but you
> are not.*

Do you think there will be a cure? And if so, when?

To be honest, this question was the reason it took me a while to respond. Something inside of me tightened when I read it. I think it's a critically important question for the Alzheimer's community as a whole to answer, especially the branches dedicated to science and research, but it feels so far from the lived experience of the disease. For folks like me, I feel there are broader questions to be asked, ones that help us exist, endure, and learn how to breathe inside the expanse of time between where we are now and a possible cure.

> " *I want us to talk about the work that needs to be done on a community level so we can ensure folks with Alzheimer's are stitched into webs of support for as long as possible.* "

I want to know about how to sustain connection with my mom as she continues to lose language.

I want to know about options for care. I want someone to ask me what my mother's name is and how my father is doing. I want us to talk about the work that needs to be done on a community level so we can ensure folks with Alzheimer's are stitched into webs of support for as long as possible. Do I also want a cure? Yes. And I also want to know how to survive until we have one.

> *Release in your mind who your loved one used to be and accept who they are today.*
>
> —J. RUSNAK, PH.D.

Enabling People with Dementia to Live Well

Cordula Dick-Muehlke, PhD

I met Cordula in California when we were both on a panel with a third speaker at an industry conference. The topic was "How Do We Provide Exceptional Dementia Care." The approach Cordula had was very different from my own approach-mine being more about creating standards of care and very objective measurements of outcomes. Hers was much more geared towards the attitudes of those in charge of the care of seniors with dementia. It made me think of the importance of that approach-can we all do better if the care and money allocated to this disease are better understood by the decision makers in both the private and public sectors? More training, more money for caregivers and possible treatment would be the likely outcomes of a trend in that direction. I tucked that in my head as I left that day and vowed to keep in touch with her.

Dr. Dick-Muehlke is a recently retired psychologist who dedicated her career to the care and support of people with Alzheimer's disease or another dementia. During her 35 years in the field, she strove to transform advance care by listening and responding to the expressed needs of those with dementia and their families as a leader, educator, and advocate.

Serving in community and academic settings, her significant contributions include heading Alzheimer's Family Services, where she led development of a state-of-the-art dementia care facility. She worked to educate innumerable families and professionals as Director of Education at the University of California Institute for Memory Impairments and Neurological Disorders (UCI MIND), and co-directed the Spirituality and Aging Certificate Program offered through New Theological Seminary of the West (NTSW). She was recognized as the 2011 Dementia Care Professional of the Year by the Alzheimer's Foundation of America. An impassioned advocate, she served as the Chair of the California Alzheimer's Disease and Related Disorders Advisory Committee, the President of the California Association of Adult Day Services, and a member of the California Alzheimer's Disease State Plan Task Force. She has contributed to a number of peer-reviewed journal articles and served as the primary editor of Psychosocial Studies of the Individual's Changing Perspectives in Alzheimer's Disease, published in 2015. Dr. Dick-Muehlke received her doctorate in clinical psychology from Fuller Graduate School of Psychology in 1993.

What advice would you give to the loved ones of someone newly diagnosed?

At times it amazes me how much advice is now readily available via a multitude of sources for people with Alzheimer's disease or another dementia and their families compared to 38 years ago when I began working in the field. Admittedly, significant gaps in access to information and support continue to exist among those who are disenfranchised in our society due to their cultural background, sexual orientation, and socioeconomic or educational status. Often left with only a diagnosis and prescription in hand from a busy physician, people with dementia and caregivers yearn for more guidance. And yet, when guidance is given, many fail to follow through with recommen-dations that could improve their lives.

So, the first thing those of us involved in sup-porting people with Alzheimer's disease or another dementia and their families must do is refrain from giving advice and listen. Advice given outside the context of the family's unique situation is advice that is unlikely to be followed. It is only when we understand what the diagnosis and its implications mean to the person affected and family that we can shape a response which resonates with their experience. What factors are influencing the diag-nosed individual's and family's interpretation of the diagnosis? The still predominant view in our society of dementia as a tragic, devastating condition for which 'nothing can be done?' Culturally rooted misperceptions of dementia as due to normal aging, mental illness, fate (i.e., one's karma), or accultura-tion stress? Past experiences with family or friends affected by dementia? Spiritual perspectives (e.g., belief in a benevolent vs. punishing God)? Such influencing factors drive the thoughts, feelings, and actions—for better or worse—of persons with dementia and their families.

> " *So, the first thing those of us involved in supporting people with Alzheimer's disease or another dementia and their families must do is refrain from giving advice and listen.* "

Most diagnosed individuals and their families view dementia through multiple lenses. Listening enables us to step into the worldview of those we seek to support (i.e., empathize) and discover what is important for them now and in the future. If we are truly committed to shifting the culture of dementia care from paternalistic to person-centered, our responses to the newly diagnosed and their families must be guided by what we have 'heard' through our ears, eyes, mind, heart, and close attention.

Do you think there will be a cure? And if so, when?

Given the current press for a cure for Alzheimer's disease and other dementias, it may be a little 'heretical' to reject this emphasis and invitation to engage in the popular game of guessing how probable it is that a cure will be found.

Don't take me wrong. Yes, I hope for and support better ways to treat and prevent Alzheimer's disease. Yet given the complexity of the dementias that science continues to reveal, it would be foolish to try and predict when a cure will emerge. As each door closes within the scientific pursuit of a cure, another one opens, and much is yet to be learned. Even as clinical trials fail, hope is warranted.

It is of greater concern for me that the widespread anxieties about developing Alzheimer's disease or another in our society—and our overall avoidance of death—feeds the hopelessness and stigma associated with cognitive decline. During an interview with *People* magazine in 2013, Pat Summit, the well-known University of Kentucky basketball coach who died of Alzheimer's disease three years later, reminded us, 'Above all, I know that Alzheimer's has brought me to a place that I was going to arrive at someday anyway. With or without this diagnosis, I was going to experience diminishment. We all do. [And] I know God doesn't take things away to be cruel. He takes things away to lighten us. He takes things away so that we can fly.'

In striving for a cure, we risk leaving behind and devaluing the 5.8 million Americans affected with Alzheimer's disease today and their families. In the words of one person with Alzheimer's disease, who echoes the feelings of many I've known, 'There is life after Alzheimer's disease.' Living well in the context of a serious illness—Alzheimer's disease or another—deserves at least equal attention to finding a cure. Enabling people with dementia to live well is as important and deserving an endeavor as the next clinical trial, and the next, and the next.

From a spiritual perspective, our current focus on a cure makes me ponder what life would be like if we eradicated suffering—whether of Alzheimer's disease or other serious and often equally heart-breaking conditions. Our spiritual traditions teach us that the suffering we all experience in one form, or another has the power to transform us into better people. Like the caregiver who participated in a support group I ran many years ago told me, 'I wouldn't wish it [dementia] on anyone, but it has made me a better person.' While having spent my career trying to lessen the suffering of people with Alzheimer's disease or another dementia and their families,

I also certainly wouldn't be the person I have become had they never entered my life. Over the past 35 years, they have gifted me with the wisdom that came from suffering alongside them, hand in hand, stretching me to grow in compassion and understanding. Wayne Ewing, an Episcopal priest, shared the experience of caring for his wife, Ann, who developed Alzheimer's disease at age 55, in the book, *Tears in God's Bottle*. In reflecting on the progression of her dementia, he noted, 'I began to ask myself, could it be that, as mystics of all spiritual traditions suggest, one's loss of time and space is really a foreshadowing of an entry into the eternal?'

Even as we seek to support people with dementia in the passage from life to death, perhaps they are truly our guides into a deeper understanding of the possibilities that the challenges of aging and our eventual death offer even in the face of Alzheimer's disease or another dementia.

It is of greater concern for me that the widespread anxieties about developing Alzheimer's disease or another in our society—and our overall avoidance of death—feeds the hopelessness and stigma associated with cognitive decline.

No matter who you are, what you've accomplished, what your financial situation is—when you're dealing with a parent with Alzheimer's, you yourself feel helpless. The parent can't work, can't live alone, and is totally dependent, like a toddler. As the disease unfolds, you don't know what to expect.

—MARIA SHRIVER

Use All of the Tools Available

PeiPei Wishnow, PhD

A scientist, entrepreneur, and healthy-aging advocate, not to mention a fellow Boston area resident, Dr. Peipei Wishnow founded Interceuticals over 20 years ago in order to create clinically tested supplements for those who want to age vibrantly, confidently, and naturally. It was suggested to me that I watch one of her presentations on the relationship between nutrition and brain aging, which was fascinating. After I did, I contacted her and had a lively conversation on the subject.

As you will see, her approach is based on a deep knowledge of Chinese Traditional Medicine and its beneficial chemical components derived from natural herbs and medicines. She is focused on bringing the best of both Western scientific methodology and Eastern holistic knowledge to the better-aging products she develops. This

53

knowledge is coupled with degrees in Science and Genetics from Zhejiang University, a PhD in Biology from CUNY and postdoctoral research at MIT and Caltech. East truly meets west.

A passionate advocate for vibrant and confident aging, she is a skilled public speaker and spokesperson.

What advice would you give to the loved ones of someone newly diagnosed?

To a person or their family newly diagnosed with Alzheimer's I would say: 'Be open. Search for products and service es that have solid clinical backing and try them but don't limit yourself to only Western medical treatments.' Use all of the tools available to help you or your loved ones, don't wait for the arrival of one miracle drug. Take whatever can help. Even if an available treatment can't reverse or completely stop the disease progression, any slowing of that progression or improvements of the quality of life both for the patients and caregivers is a huge plus.

The current scientific understanding of the human brain is still very limited. I believe we will see not only more and more breakthrough discoveries in neuroscience but also a profound new understanding of some time-tested healing wisdom.

> *Use all of the tools available to help you or your loved ones, don't wait for the arrival of one miracle drug.*

Do you think there will be a cure? And if so, when?

I believe there will be a cure in the future, perhaps in 5-10 years, as scientists understand more about human brain, its structure and functions. Or this dreadful disease will be transformed into a much more humanely manageable aging issue, not as painful and costly as it is now. I do believe prevention of dementia will be one of the keys for the future. If you look around, this transition is happening even as we speak with the integration of healthy lifestyle, proper exercise, quality sleep, and well-rounded nutrition.

"I do believe prevention of dementia will be one of the keys for the future."

In generations past, the world came together to take on the great killers. We have stood against malaria, cancer, HIV, and AIDS— and we are just as resolute today. I want December 11, 2013, to go down as the day that the global fight began.

—FORMER BRITISH PRIME MINISTER DAVID CAMERON

Own the Disease

Mal Allard

Mal Allard is a Licensed Nurse and Alzheimer's and Dementia Consultant, and a respected and thoughtful author and lecturer on Alzheimer's and related dementias. She has an almost intuitive grasp of the affect it has on those diagnosed and, almost as importantly, on those that love them. I have heard her speak many times, and always felt that her warmth and relatability, along with her intimate knowledge of the day-to-day lives of the seniors and their families on the journey, brings comfort to all who know her.

Her kind and timely advice has eased many a family's burdens, and she has trained innumerable people in the field as to how to best care for those seniors who depend on us, while keeping their dignity firmly intact. In 2003, Mal founded and developed Their Real World, an Alzheimer's and Dementia company providing education for professionals, family caregivers, and the community at large. Mal is currently developing an Alzheimer's and Dementia professionals workshop entitled: "An Alzheimer's Whisperer."

▨ What advice would you give to the loved ones of someone newly diagnosed?

I would advise the newly diagnosed person to:

1. Be yourself. Be present. Own the disease. Make a difference.
2. Never be embarrassed by your forgetfulness or confusion.
3. Share your true emotion. Find moments of positivity.
4. Seek support of those who are also on the journey—they need you.
5. Keep your sense of humor. Give yourself a pat on the back.

And I would advise a loved one of a newly diagnosed person to:

1. Listen to them and let them be present. Their emotions are telling you something.

2. Find the positive within the journey for the both of you– your person is still present.
3. Help them to live a seemingly normal life within their dementia.
4. Put all things in perspective. Take care of you, too! Learn, share, and seek support.
5. Keep your sense of humor. Give yourself a pat on the back.

> *" Never be embarrassed by your forgetfulness or confusion. "*

Do you think there will be a cure? And if so, when?

Yes, I believe there will be a cure; I need to have that concerted hope to do what I've been doing for all these years. If the cure cannot be yesterday or today—then praying for tomorrow.

> *" If the cure cannot be yesterday or today—then praying for tomorrow. "*

It's shameful. You don't want to talk about the fact that your parents have Alzheimer's. Another reason is the patients themselves are demented; they can't advocate for themselves. There isn't a Michael J. Fox equivalent for Alzheimer's.

—SETH ROGEN

I suffer from short-term memory loss. It runs in my family. At least I think it does... where are they?

—DORY from Disney's *Finding Nemo*

Living Moment
By Moment

Jolene Brakey

Jolene Brakey, author, speaker, and trainer extraordinaire, was one of the first people I met, over 25 years ago, who opened my eyes to the fact that we, as senior living professionals, were largely thinking of our programming for people with dementia the way we might think of doing it with young school children. We responsibly enough kept them active and engaged in things like crafts and puzzles. But we were, back in the early to late 90's, more concerned with activities that produced something we could proudly display for the families of our residents. "Look what your mother made today" when we in fact had "helped" quite a bit. Her philosophy, borne from a combination of insight and first-hand knowledge gained as a dementia program professional, was quite different. Her method, as her first book advocates, was to remind us that we may not be able to create perfectly wonderful days for our residents, Alzheimer's does not allow that, but we can create perfectly wonderful moments is filled with joy, for the joy is in how the experience makes us feel, not in the end product.

I absorbed her method, first reading her helpful and aptly titled book "Creating Moments of Joy" which is a beloved best seller, now on its fifth edition, and which has since become a bible for activity directors at dementia care communities everywhere. I was so impressed by the refreshing attitude and respect for the residents that her approach demonstrated that I hired her to train our staff and address families at one of our communities. Watching her teach was so enlightening—you could see the light dawn on the staff as to what truly mattered—not what the result was but the emotion of the moment, the light in the resident's eyes, the feeling of normality and inclusivity. As I created some of my own specialty dementia programs, such as a unique cooking experience called "Memory Making Baking," I kept that concept firmly in mind.

I reconnected with her recently, and she was taking a year off to do as she often advises, "I am living moment by moment." Simple to say, but so difficult to do at

times; her insights embody this commonsense approach,
developed over the past twenty-five plus years and aimed
at keeping the joy in lives no matter what their diagnoses.

What advice would you give to the loved ones of someone newly diagnosed?

The person with dementia is always your teacher in the moment. To try to figure it out or project into the future is insanity.

Do you think there will be a cure? And if so, when?

The 'cure' to any disease is accepting the person as they are right now.

> *As the sixth leading cause of death, Alzheim-*
> *er's disease is the only cause of death in the*
> *top 10 that we currently do not have a way to*
> *prevent, or to stop or slow its progression.*
>
> —HEATHER SNYDER, PHD,
> director of medical and scientific operations
> at the Alzheimer's Association

We Are Not Losing the Person

Teepa Snow

Teepa Snow is another of those people who opened my eyes to the way we all can best interact in a therapeutic and genuine way with those we care for who have Alzheimer's and other memory loss. Her boundless energy, witnessed first-hand during the many training seminars our company hired her for, provide inspiration for people involved in caregiving for those with Alzheimer's all around the world. I first met her 18 years ago when she was just starting to make a name for herself with her nearly revolutionary approach to training caregivers. She is able to grab your attention and hold you riveted for the entire interactive presentation. She is always urging listeners to learn how to re-energize the care given, so these seniors can thrive as much as possible on their journey.

Teepa Snow is an occupational therapist by trade with over forty years of clinical practice experience. She is one of the world's leading educators on dementia and the care that accompanies it. In 2005, she founded Positive Approach® to Care (PAC), a company that provides dementia care training, services, and products around the world. Her GEMS program is in widespread use, and she is active internationally as well. Her new book, Understanding the Changing Brain *is the first in a planned series, and a must-read.*

What advice would you give to the loved ones of someone newly diagnosed?

I would say that people are precious and in the right setting can still shine. We are not losing the person; they're still there, but we need to modify our expectations and the setting. Your brain works better than their brain; you need to figure out how to interact—you can change the environment, the task, or your own behavior. Remember—dementia doesn't rob a person of their dignity, it's our reaction to them that does.

Remember—dementia doesn't rob a person of their dignity, it's our reaction to them that does.

Do you think there will be a cure? And if so, when?

The United States isn't prepared for the growing number of elderly who will suffer from Alzheimer's within the next decade. More than 5 million Americans now have the disease and within 10 years, nearly 13 1/2 million Americans could be living with it, unless a cure is found. We're about to hit the baby boomers, and we really don't have a plan that works. We're nowhere near where we need to be at this time to deal with it. We also have the problem that this disease spans eight to 12 years on average.

It's the third most expensive disease to have, but it's at the bottom of the barrel for reimbursement. Most of Alzheimer's expenses are out-of-the-pocket, and incontinence products alone will put a family in debt, let alone sitter service or support service or community living.

I always say, 'Until there's a cure, there's care.'

> *"We're nowhere near where we need to be at this time to deal with it."*

There are only four kinds of people in the world. Those who have been caregivers. Those who are currently caregivers. Those who will be caregivers, and those who will need a caregiver.

—ROSALYN CARTER

No One Size Fits All

Elizabeth Cobbs, MD

Dr. Cobbs is an influential internist, geriatrician and palliative care doctor with GW Medical Faculty Associates and a professor of medicine at The George Washington School of Medicine and Health Sciences. She has over 41 years of experience in the medical field. Since 2011, she has been chief of Geriatrics, Extended Care and Palliative Care at the Washington DC VA Medical Center. She serves as Associate Editor of the Journal of the American Geriatrics Society, among her many other endeavors.

I was introduced to Elizabeth as a result of my work in Washington, DC with the first all affordable assisted living community in Ward seven, and only the second one in the district. She came to me well recommended, and after speaking with her I quickly understood why. She combines her wide-ranging experience and education with

a passion to get it right for seniors, especially those dealing
with dementia on top of the normal challenges of aging.

What advice would you give to the loved ones of someone newly diagnosed?

I always try to find out what their experience with the disease is, what do they already know. To me that is the epitome of truly person-centered care, to understand their circumstances individually as there is no one size fits all. Sometimes they know a great deal about Alzheimer's because they have cared for another family member with the disease. If not, I fill in the knowledge gaps.

> **We are learning more about how to delay the progression, particularly there are many powerful lifestyle interventions that can delay the progression of functional decline.**

Secondly, I talk about the incredible times we are living in, where we now have an opportunity to live a long life with chronic conditions that used to be death sentences, but now we often can live comfortably with them or a long time. We are learning more about how to delay the progression, particularly there are many powerful lifestyle interventions that can delay the progression of functional decline. Here we are living in 2022, and the health literacy of the person and the family has grown. Peoples' belief systems are not transparent, so we need to understand what they want and believe in order to offer appropriate hope.

Do you think there will be a cure? And if so, when?

I think the question, more accurately, should be, 'Will there be an effective disease modifying therapy?' I believe that is certainly within our grasp. Maybe it will be in the form of blood pressure control, maybe it will be diet or exercise related. It hurts me to see the desire for a pharmacological drug expected for everything that ails you. As far as environment, I am glad we are investing in age friendly cities instead of nursing homes.

I think the question, more accurately, should be, 'Will there be an effective disease modifying therapy?'

Dementia is the biggest health and social care challenge of our generation, but research into the condition has been hugely underfunded. This lack of funding has hampered progress and also restricted the number of scientists and clinicians working in the dementia field.

—JAMES PICKETT, head of research at the UK's Alzheimer's Society

The Difference Between Providing Care and Providing Treatment

Judy Cornish

*Judy Cornish is an author, founder of the Dementia &
Alzheimer's Wellbeing Network (DAWN®), creator of
the DAWN Method® of dementia care, and a retired
elder law attorney. Her two books,* The Dementia Handbook *and* Dementia with Dignity, *take
person-centered dementia care from theory to practice
by identifying the skills not lost to dementia. Through
DAWN, Cornish provides online training programs for
families and professional caregivers, as well as certifica-
tion courses for agencies and facilities.*

*I was thoroughly impressed with the level of detail
contained in her books and was thrilled when she agreed
to provide a quote for my book, as I knew it would be
as thoughtful as she is. Cornish's life work has been to*

make dignified dementia care and aging in place available for all.

What advice would you give to the loved ones of someone newly diagnosed?

My advice to those who receive a diagnosis of dementia—or have a loved one who has been diagnosed—is to come to grips with the difference between providing care and providing treatment. Focusing on diagnosis and treatment is only helpful when there are interventions that can return the person to health.

When someone is diagnosed with cancer, we turn to doctors for help because there are effective treatments for cancer. We rightly focus on obtaining an accurate diagnosis and identifying potential treatments because knowing the type of cancer and its treatment options increases the likelihood of recovery and cure—of the person's eventual return to health.

However, when there is no treatment or cure and the person must live with a condition, where is the benefit in continuing with a medical model? It makes more sense to turn to a care model.

Now, instead of focusing on ways to return the person to health (treatment), we focus on maximizing their comfort and quality of life (care). We put our efforts into identifying and meeting their changing needs, and away from tabulating the ways in which their condition or behavior has become abnormal. We turn our hopes away from seeing them regain health, toward seeing them respond to our efforts at reestablishing companionship and comfort. Providing care is the opposite of providing treatment.

When we understand that our role as the companions of people who are experiencing dementia is to learn how to better support their new emotional needs and changing skills, there is less stress for both parties and companionship and quality of life can return. There is peace in recognizing this difference.

“When there is no treatment or cure and the person must live with a condition, where is the benefit in continuing with a medical model? It makes more sense to turn to a care model.”

Do you think there will be a cure? And if so, when?

No doubt there will eventually be medications that prove reliable in slowing or improving the symptoms of Alzheimer's disease. However, I don't think we will ever succeed in curing dementia itself. I believe we will always have people who are experiencing dementia, and that we should embrace learning how to better live *with* dementia, as we will always have it in our families and communities.

We still sometimes think of Alzheimer's as a synonym for dementia, even though it is not. Dementia is a progressive condition that can result from a number of diseases—including Parkinson's and cardiovascular disease—and may follow physical events, such as a bad reaction to anesthetic or chemo, even an earlier-in-life traumatic brain injury. Lifestyle choices also affect the likelihood of developing dementia. We know that sedentary people are more likely to experience it than active people, while lifetime learners and those whose diets are higher in natural foods than processed foods are less likely.

> *I believe we will always have people who are experiencing dementia, and that we should embrace learning how to better live with dementia, as we will always have it in our families and communities.*

To my mind, we won't see dementia cured until we see food corporations designing food for nutritive value and digestibility rather than for shelf life and transportability; until we see employers equally as concerned about their employees' health as their shareholders' profits; and until we as a nation begin prioritizing quality of life for all over unfettered material gain for some.

Being deeply loved by someone gives you strength, while loving someone deeply gives you courage.

—LAO TZU

The Journey is a Process

Kelly McCarthy

Kelly has written a book for caregivers, but most importantly, she has truly devoted her career to helping improve the lives of seniors with memory loss, and she does it in such an uplifting, caring and joyful way that I just had to include her perspective.

Her book, Brass Ring Memoirs, consists of encouraging stories and uses tried and true practical methods to help caregivers in their demanding roles. Her methods led to a training program that she employs to help professional caregivers learn the most updated methods of care as they help seniors on their journeys. She is currently Vice President of Resident Engagement and Memory Care Services at The Northbridge Companies, where she makes a difference every day.

What advice would you give to the loved ones of someone newly diagnosed?

The first thing I always ask is how are you? This allows them to process their own feelings and will help support the emotions surrounding the diagnosis. Then I would ask what questions they have. Starting the conversation by asking what it is they want to know or what is their understanding will give a person the starting point to focus. Narrowing down the topics is helpful, instead of just talking about things they haven't even thought about yet, which may be scary and overwhelming. The journey is a process so the final thing I would say is to encourage them to join a support group. We are both teachers and students during this journey, and groups can be a great way to get and give support.

Starting the conversation by asking what it is they want to know or what is their understanding will give a person the starting point to focus.

Do you think there will be a cure? And if so, when?

I will always have hope. As for the timing, I will say that I hope in my lifetime we get closer. I hope there are medications and non-pharmacological approaches to stop dementia from occurring. Very much like the success we see with Human Immunodeficiency Virus, HIV and how it has slowed and diminished the occurrence of full-blown Acquired Immune Deficiency Syndrome, AIDS. It would be great to hear a person say someday 'I have Alzheimer's, but I do not have dementia' . . . I'll take that.

" *I will always have hope.* "

Hope is being able to see that there is light in all of the darkness.
—DESMUND TUTU

There Are Still Lots of Things That Can Be Done

Dr. Emerson Lombardo

Dr. Lombardo is the President and Founder of the Brain Health and Wellness Center® and Adjunct Research Assistant Professor of Neurology at the Boston University School of Medicine. She is also an Alzheimer's researcher with the Boston University Alzheimer's Disease Center. Nancy is a co-founder of both the Alzheimer's Association and Alzheimer's Disease International and formerly served on the Medical and Scientific Advisory Committee of the Massachusetts/New Hampshire chapter of the Alzheimer's Association.

    I met Nancy several years ago when I was working on developing a better diet for our assisted living residents at the company I work for. I had learned that diet was such an important part of our well-being and wanted our seniors to have the best shot at staving off the many effects of a poor diet for as long as possible, not to mention helping a new generation, namely our staff, to understand the importance of diet in successful ageing. We already had a successful Eat Fresh/Eat Local dining program but wanted to add science to our selections.

I did not have to look far, for right in Massachusetts was an internationally acclaimed Alzheimer's researcher who had developed her own Brain Health and Wellness program that we soon aligned ourselves with. We had a wonderful time working with her team to find the "sweet spot" if you will indulge me in a pun, between what were the healthiest snacks and what the residents will enjoy— they were not always identical, and with the cooperation of a group of our chefs led by Chef Jason Wallin and Chef Jamie Bell, we found what worked and served them to our delighted residents. Along the way, we learned so much about how brain health and heart health are happily aligned, making the knowledge gained do double duty for our overall health.

What advice would you give to the loved ones of someone newly diagnosed?

I do often meet people who are newly diagnosed, or sometimes I am asked to speak at a support group and one of the things that I tell them is that there are still lots of things that can be done to slow the advance of the disease and they are well worth trying.

I give them my five most important lifestyle tips. First of all, I tell them that if there's just one thing you could do it would be to improve their nutritional intake, and the best thing to do in that regard is to cut out sugary foods as much as possible. The science behind this suggestion is that sugar is shown to be responsible for an inflammatory effect which is detrimental to your brain. Sugar causes an increase of one of the two pathological proteins, beta amyloid, that in excess kills brain cells. There's really nothing good about sugar for your body and if people still crave sweetness, I recommend they eat whole fruits, or add cinnamon to foods if they like cinnamon.

My other dietary recommendation is to reduce the amount of red meat in their diet. Eating red meat once a week is not going to hurt, but for reasons that are not fully understood a lot of red meat is detrimental for your health; red meat also increases buildup of the harmful beta amyloid in the brain (and pork along with beef and lamb is a "red" meat). Fish is a much better choice especially those that are high in omega-3's. And poultry is better for us than red meat. To help make eating pleasurable, as well as brain healthier, another important thing is to increase the intake of vegetables, especially green leafy vegetables. If people say they don't like cooked greens, I always suggest they add herbal condiments they like such as mustard, vinegar, and/or hot spices.

Herbs and spices are a spectacular way to increase brain health antioxidants/nutrients concentrated in small volumes since they taste so good. I often recommend Trader Joe's 21 Seasoning Salute which is salt free but full of herbs, and inexpensive too. Starting an herb garden is a great way to get them fresh and enjoy the pleasure of growing your own food.

The second brain healthy lifestyle is exercise. Even if there are mobility issues, you can move your arms with a good, seated workout. This helps to speed up the creation of what we call baby brain cells in the hippocampus as well as keep your heart and blood vessels healthy, which helps the brain.

My third recommendation, which also helps the new brain cells get integrated into the brain, is to keep on doing things that stimulate the brain, like meeting and talking to new people, being involved with pleasurable activities, things that create new experiences rather than sitting and watching television.

Fourth, keep socially engaged with other people; not only does this usually help your mood, but it is very stimulating for your brain. So, if you can exercise with other people, you get a 'two-for.' Since music is great for the brain, dancing gives you multiple benefits.

The fifth thing is sleep. We have come a long way in being able to help seniors who notoriously have problems with sleep to make it more attainable for them. For example, there are herbs that help along with medical sleep clinics.

> *First of all, I tell them that if there's just one thing you could do it would be to improve their nutritional intake, and the best thing to do in that regard is to cut out sugary foods as much as possible.*

Do you think there will be a cure? And if so, when?

As far as 'will there be a cure,' that is a difficult question because if there *is* a cure, it will probably look different than what people are now expecting. It will probably be a combination of medicine and lifestyle changes, and ideally will be tailored to everyone. 'Precision medicine' is coming to brain health and Alzheimer's prevention. Medical doctors who are independent researchers and work closely with patients are definitely pushing the FDA and drug companies to look into using bio markers to become part of outcome measurements in major clinical trials because the cognitive tests that they have used in the past are not always sensitive enough because of the variety of ways that cognition declines and varies during the day or month. I will say that I do feel that there will be a breakthrough even though many drug companies have given up the chase for a cure because they have come to realize how very complex this disease is.

I am heartened to know that the 'worldwide 'FINGER" initiative studying how the brain healthy lifestyles I've just listed involves 45 countries in early 2022, all cooperating and sharing (and improving) research methods, data and results. This effort is coordinated and funded by our U.S. Alzheimer's Association.

> *As far as "will there be a cure," that is a difficult question because if there is a cure, it will probably look different than what people are now expecting.*

*While the final chapter of my life with
dementia may be trying, nothing has diminished my gratitude and deep appreciation for
the countless blessings in my life.*

—SANDRA DAY O'CONNOR

A Diagnosis of Dementia Should Not Be Viewed As the End of Life

Josh Freitas

I have gone to more industry seminars and conferences over the years than I care to count, including many on dementia. Most times I come away disappointed, as the information is merely already known ideas and techniques rehashed in a not very innovative or helpful way. However, when I went to a session led by Josh, I did something uncharacteristic for me. I stayed after the talk and went up to talk to him, so taken by the fresh approach and insight he exhibited. I followed his career path and enjoyed his books.

Joshua J. Freitas is an award-winning memory care program developer, researcher, and author. His care and training philosophies have been featured in prominent publications nationally. Freitas serves as the Vice

President of Program Development at CERTUS Senior Living where he oversees memory care philosophy and initiatives throughout the company.

Currently, Freitas is also a Doctoral student at the California Institute of Integral Studies where he focuses on Transformative Gerontology and Aging Neuroscience. Freitas holds five certifications related to dementia care. His two recent book publications, "The Dementia Concept" and "Joining Grandma's Journey," aim to change the way society views individuals who are living with Alzheimer's disease. Enjoy his thoughtful answers and consider reading his books!

What advice would you give to the loved ones of someone newly diagnosed?

A diagnosis of dementia should not be viewed as the end of life. People can live with dementia for up to thirty years. We must empower people with dementia to continue to live purposefully. One major challenge is to educate the general public, healthcare providers, and medical personnel not to perpetuate the stigmas associated with dementia. We have the potential to improve quality of life through non-pharmacological, compensatory strategies for interaction. Although there is no cure for Alzheimer's disease or related dementia, in most cases there is a great deal that can be done to help people live active and fulfilling lives for a longer period of time.

Through a combination of pharmacological and non-pharmacological interventions, we can help people sustain awareness and promote neuroplasticity. Doing so naturally elevates mood, reinforces skills, and increases confidence. Neuroplasticity also reinforces the hippocampus, which is the part of the brain that directs memory, enabling people to create new memories and retain them longer.

Many people who are diagnosed with dementia express fear of losing their independence. For many years, the dementia care community has overlooked the right of those with dementia to be active participants in their own care. More and more individuals are coming forward and demanding to have a say in what happens throughout the course of their dementia progression.

When all medical decisions are made by a healthcare proxy and all financial decisions are made by the individual's Power of Attorney, this takes away the choice and the voice of individuals with dementia.

To counteract this problem, the Alzheimer's Bill of Rights has been drafted to help people with dementia to foster a sense of independence. This Bill of Rights strongly reinforces their rights to be informed of their condition, given opportunities for engagement, and given a sense of independence within a safe, structured, and predictable environment.

The care we provide must uphold these values. We must recognize the importance of engaging with the individual and making them a vital participant in their own healing.

> *Although there is no cure for Alzheimer's disease or related dementia, in most cases there is a great deal that can be done to help people live active and fulfilling lives for a longer period of time.*

Do you think there will be a cure? And if so, when?

Many researchers say that there is no cure in sight, and each year the number of cases grows worldwide. It is an epidemic that is soon to be classified as a pandemic. If a cure is not found within the next few decades, the rising cost of care could cripple the economy, and people living with dementia will suffer from a lack of funding for treatment options and caregiver education.

Fortunately, there is something that we can do to combat this problem through our work as caregivers. By increasing public awareness and improving caregiver education, we can help eliminate some of the detrimental stigmas associated with dementia. We must join the movement to change the way people with dementia and memory impairment are viewed and treated. In return, individuals with dementia can sustain and increase engagement with their lives.

> *By increasing public awareness and improving caregiver education, we can help eliminate some of the detrimental stigmas associated with dementia.*

> *Caregiving often calls us to lean into love we didn't know possible.*
> —TIA WALKER

Have Hope

Karen Hoglund

Karen is one of my oldest and dearest friends, going back to when we were both kids growing up in a small Massachusetts town. We were soon both young brides trying to figure out how to be mothers, wives and still have a life of our own. Over the years we have shared joys and sorrows, and sadly one of those sorrows for Karen was a parent diagnosed with Alzheimer's. She and I talked often about how this affected her, her family, and her understanding of the disease. Her always honest answers are included here to give a glimpse into how this disease affects families firsthand.

What advice would you give to the loved ones of someone newly diagnosed?

If I met a friend in the grocery store and found out her parent had just been diagnosed with Alzheimer's, this is what I would tell her:

- Treat your parent with dignity. They *will* feel it.
- Hug them often, hold their hand, it will feel familiar to them.
- Talk to them with respect. They are still your parent.
- If they express ideas or plans, don't tell them they can't do that, instead make a plan with them, and make them feel that they have worth.
- Don't correct them, they are trying to find the right words, they know there is something really wrong, but they don't know what it is. It bothers them all the time that they can't figure it out. Of course it gets frustrating.
- Help them with grooming so they look nice, it matters.
- Treat them like an adult and have lots of patience.
- Go through old photos and talk about people they remember, don't make an issue of those they don't.
- Mostly try not to correct them, try to have plenty of patience, and when they get agitated play music from their era. If they can hear it, it will settle them down.

It's a long, hard journey for everyone.

"Treat your parent with dignity."

Do you think there will be a cure? And if so, when?

I have hope that it will happen in my grandchildren's lifetime.

> One of the hardest things you will ever have
> to do my dear, is to grieve the loss of a person
> who is still alive.
>
> —ANONYMOUS

Set The Stage in The Best Possible Way for a Good Life

Stephen Gordon, MD

Dr. Gordon is a board-certified geriatrician with a lifelong passion for improving the care of the elderly. He founded Edenbridge Health in 2016 after spending two years working as a primary care geriatrician at the Program for All-Inclusive Care for the Elderly (PACE) at Upham's Corner Health Center in Dorchester, Massachusetts, as well as director of the Iora Health Fellowship in Primary Care Innovation, where he specialized in clinical systems design, care planning, and provider development. He continues to practice on a limited basis at Upham's Corner PACE. He is on the faculty of Harvard Medical School and holds clinical appointments at Beth Israel Deaconess Medical Center, Boston Medical Center, and Hebrew Senior Life, where he teaches in the Harvard

Multi-Campus Fellowship in Geriatrics. He is a supervis-
ing physician for United Community Health Plan, where
he oversees more than 30 nurse practitioners caring for
nursing home patients across the Boston area.

Stephen's career has spanned the worlds of medicine
and business. After graduating from Harvard College,
he spent four years as a consultant for the Advisory
Board Company, where he worked on issues relating
to hospital strategy and operations, including service
line growth, facility design, primary care strategy, and
physician-hospital relations. After a year at the Harvard
Interfaculty Program for Health Systems Improvement,
focusing on issues of healthcare leadership, he earned
an MBA from the Wharton School at the University of
Pennsylvania, where he double majored in health care
systems and operations. Subsequently, he attended the
Yale School of Medicine. He completed his residency
in internal medicine at Beth Israel Deaconess Medical
Center in Boston, followed by a two-year fellowship in
geriatrics at Harvard Medical School.

Stephen has consulted for the Leapfrog Group, the
Clinton Foundation, the Governments of Ukraine and
Nigeria, the City of Cape Town Clinics in South Africa,
Renaissance Health, as well as hospitals and health sys-
tems across the U.S.

What advice would you give to the loved ones of someone newly diagnosed?

When I speak to caregivers for the newly diagnosed, there are usually five points I like to make. The first and most important is to help them understand that there will be a long period of uncertainty as to how the disease will progress you don't know exactly how quickly they will progress and what stages they will go through, but you need to be prepared and always think about what the next step could be. What that means is that you're going to want to set the stage in the best possible way for a good life such as making sure the house is set up well making sure they are not lonely making sure you put long-term care in place and making sure that you have ample support for this journey.

Secondly, I would say do not spend too much time zeroing in on a specific diagnosis. Of course, first you need to make sure that you have ruled out anything reversible such as vitamin deficiency. But once those are ruled out knowing the actual diagnosis is of limited value because, unfortunately, it's not like we have great cures for them.

The third point I make is to urge them to have that end-of-life conversation with them as soon as possible this conversation is important, and it may be much harder to have if you wait due to changes in their cognitive status, they may get depressed they may have less understanding of the significance of this discussion. This is not about how you feel about how their end of life should be this is about what they want. Do they want to extend their life through extraordinary lifesaving efforts, or will they focus more on the quality of the life that they have left? Also don't forget to talk to them about how they want to be remembered and what their legacy will be. How will your celebration of their life show that earth will be different because they lived on it? Make sure they know while they are still able to understand it how important their life has been.

My fourth point involves a conversation on how to live with other health issues going forward. Do we cut your medications in half? Do we fire some of the medical specialists we are seeing? While you may want to focus on some health issues that will help their life be as good as possible, you are at the point now where you're no longer trying to extend their life beyond what is likely to happen. My suggestion is, if they always enjoyed spending time with their grandkids do that with them instead of spending time at multiple doctors' offices.

And finally, the fifth topic I bring up is to urge them to have a discussion with your medical practitioner about the Alzheimer's medications to see if they are right in your loved one's life. We know that they're not right for everybody. While it's perfectly reasonable to try them out, they are not miracles. Generally, we see that the symptoms will slow or not progress for six months at most, but you need to think about what stage you are 'freezing' them at for those six months. They can get stuck in a difficult stage of the disease where they are embarrassed by their losses and not able to enjoy life as much as if they progressed to a less stressful stage. Think this decision over, as it is not without consequences.

> *The first and most important is to help them understand that there will be a long period of uncertainty as to how the disease will progress you don't know exactly how quickly they will progress and what stages they will go through, but you need to be prepared and always think about what the next step could be.*

Do you think there will be a cure? And if so, when?

As far as a cure, I don't think there will be a cure anytime soon. We are not optimistic because the more we study it the more we have realized that this disease is significantly more complex than we originally thought and there is much more interaction between different neurological processes. I often joke that a close friend of mine is a well-known neurologist and I'm just not that impressed with how well he understands this disease process. I think he would agree!

What we do hope for and expect is that in the coming years we will find that we are able to live better lives even with this disease through research that is now going on. For that, I am hopeful.

> *We are not optimistic because the more we study it the more we have realized that this disease is significantly more complex than we originally thought and there is much more interaction between different neurological processes.*

> We could have a serious epidemic on our hands. Alzheimer's is a ticking time bomb in the heads of people in my generation. We must defuse it before it detonates and destroys our minds. Time is running out.
>
> —DAVID HYDE PIERCE, actor

The Method of Communication

Govind Bharwani, Ph.D.

Dr. Bharwini is the Co-Director of Ergonomics and Alzheimer's Care in the College of Engineering at Wright State University, and a nationally recognized expert in Alzheimer's and dementia care. He is the developer of the nationally recognized BBET Program (Behavior Based Ergonomics Therapy) through his company, DGM.

I have had the pleasure of working with Dr. Bharwani and his BBET program several times and have learned something new at every encounter. His understanding of effectively applied ergonomics and neuroscience principles make every interaction more thoughtful and effective. I personally have learned so much from his approach, and his never-ending quest to find what works for each and every participant in the BBET program, that I wanted his insight to be shared with all.

What advice would you give to the loved ones of someone newly diagnosed?

I would advise a caregiver that the major reason for mental stress between the caregiver and PWD (Person with Dementia) is as a result of the method of communication and interaction between the two. The family and or caregivers often use verbal methods of communication while the PWD prefers non-verbal methods of communication. This mis-match is the root cause of many behavior problems in Memory Care. Based on Neuroscience research, the quality of life of the PWD can be improved if caregivers learn and use the method of communication naturally preferred by the PWD. This will also help to reduce behavior problems, falls, the use of psychotropic medications, as well as caregiver stress.

Do you think there will be a cure? And if so, when?

Ah, that is the great unknown.

We don't remember days,
we remember moments.
—CESARE PAVESE

In Their Own Words: Thoughts From Those on the Journey

*You have to be patient with [Alzheimer's].
Once you understand that it's a medical
condition, you become a little more
compassionate. You get less frustrated.*

—KIM CAMPBELL, WIFE OF
SINGER GLEN CAMPBELL

IN 2017, THE NATIONAL treasure, singer Glen Campbell, died of Alzheimer's. His family revealed his Alzheimer's diagnosis in 2011. While he was still able to communicate, the "Rhinestone Cowboy" singer became an advocate for funding for the prevention and cure of the disease. To that end,

Campbell traveled to Capitol Hill in 2012, along with his wife and children Ashley, Cal and Shannon. Sadly, by early 2014, Campbell's Alzheimer's had progressed to the point where it was no longer safe for him to remain in his home, and he was moved to a facility to receive full-time care.

> *Alzheimer's is brutal. I mean, it's associated with losing your memory, but you don't just forget who people are; you also forget how to talk, how to eat, how to do everything. That's hard to wrap your head around until you actually see it.*
>
> —SETH ROGEN

In an essay for InStyle published in 2017, Seth Rogen explained that his now-wife, Lauren Miller, found out her mom had early-onset Alzheimer's disease less than a year after they started dating. Rogen said he was "shocked" by what happened to her as a result of the disease. The couple founded Hilarity for Charity, a nonprofit organization that raises money for Alzheimer's disease and caregiver resources, though he said his ultimate goal is "to make the organization obsolete."

> *I think this whole issue, whether it's
> Alzheimer's or caregiving, has a long way to
> go, I think, as a national conversation. What
> do caregivers need? What do they look like?
> What do we as a country need? Why are
> two-thirds of the Alzheimer's cases women?*
>
> —MARIA SHRIVER

Inspired by her father, former First Lady of California, Maria Shriver, is a staunch advocate for Alzheimer's disease through her nonprofit, Shriver Report, and has also written a children's book and produced films about Alzheimer's disease.

> *For baby boomers, I feel like the canary in
> the coal mine while scientists search for a
> cure. I fear the day when I put my fingers
> on the keyboard and don't know how to
> write anymore.*
>
> —GREG O'BRIEN

An investigative journalist living on Cape Cod, Greg decided to take control of his own story after his Alzheimer's diagnosis in 2009 at age 59. He wrote a book called "On Pluto: Inside the Mind of Alzheimer's" about what it feels like to undergo the beginning stages of dementia. He later wrote an essay for The Washington Post detailing some of the changes he has noticed in his mind and urging others to keep up the fight. "By documenting Alzheimer's, I'm getting even with it," he wrote.

> *While the final chapter of my life with dementia may be trying, nothing has diminished my gratitude and deep appreciation for the countless blessings in my life.*
>
> —SANDRA DAY-O'CONNOR
> wrote in a letter released by
> the Supreme Court's public
> information office.

In October 2018, retired Supreme Court Justice Sandra Day-O'Connor revealed that she was in the "beginning stages of dementia, probably Alzheimer's disease." She said she would continue to live in

Phoenix but would be stepping away from public life. Tragically, her husband John also had Alzheimer's, which according to a new biography was part of the reason why she retired from the Supreme Court in 2005. Her son, Jay, wrote that when she was first diagnosed, his mother didn't want to believe it—her worst fear—given a family history of dementia. So, for a number of years, "She just tried to power through. She's a woman who has been able to overcome so many powerful obstacles in her life and career. And it turns out that dementia and Alzheimer's is just the obstacle you can't overcome."

> *Alzheimer's is me, unwinding, losing trust in myself, a butt of my own jokes and on bad days capable of playing hunt the slipper by myself and losing. You can't battle it; you can't be a plucky 'survivor.' It steals you from yourself.*
>
> —TERRY PRATCHETT

Author Terry Pratchett was diagnosed with posterior cortical atrophy (PCA) in 2007. PCA is believed to be either a form of Alzheimer's disease or possibly a unique disease. Before his death in 2015, he wrote an essay published by the Alzheimer's Society and later in The Guardian reflecting on his diagnosis. He described PCA as having "extreme problems handling the physical world," but still being able to "talk your way out of it." He also expressed his belief that one day there would be a cure. "It is a physical disease, not a mystic curse; therefore, it will fall to a physical cure. There's time to kill the demon before it grows," he wrote.

> *It is a strange, sad irony that so often, in the territory of a disease that robs an individual of memory, caregivers are often the forgotten.*
>
> —KAREN WILDER

Gene Wilder was famously quiet about his Alzheimer's diagnosis, but in 2018, 15 months after his death, his widow Karen wrote a powerful essay about their marriage and his final years of life. She explained how physically, and emotionally taxing Alzheimer's can be on caregivers and urged researchers not to forget their needs too.

The Alzheimer's Association in the United
States, founded by Jerome Stone, found
me because they had heard rumors that my
mom [Rita Hayworth] was diagnosed. Jerry
says, "We're a small family group, and we
would like to know if you'd like to join us and
spread the word about this disease.' I said,
'Absolutely.'

—YASMIN AGA KHAN

As an iconic beauty of the decade, Rita Hayworth was one of the most popular pin-up girls for GIs during World War II. Her career started as a backup dancer in the 1926 short film La Fiesta, and she would eventually star in 61 films before finally retiring in 1972. After displaying dementia-like symptoms for over a decade, Rita was diagnosed with Alzheimer's disease in 1980 before passing away in 1987. Her death helped spread awareness of the disease which was relatively unknown by most of the public at that time. Her daughter and caretaker, Yasmin Aga Khan, served on the Board of Directors for Alzheimer's and

Related Disorders Association in addition to being the president of Alzheimer's Disease International.

> *Here is a woman who has made her husband's life her career. She has devoted herself to making Ronald Reagan's life perfect, [but] no matter what she does now, his life will never be perfect again.*
>
> —FRED RYAN, former presidential aide

As her husband's condition worsened, the famous woman-behind-the-man found herself cast in a challenging and unexpected supporting role. Former President Ronald Reagan's response to his Alzheimer's diagnosis was to sit down and write a letter to his fellow Americans. In it, he said he was sharing his diagnosis to encourage a "clearer understanding" of the people affected by it and acknowledged that families often bear a "heavy burden." In his words: "I intend to live the remainder of the years God gives me on this earth doing the things I have always done. I only wish there was some way I could spare Nancy from this painful experience. When the time comes, I am confident that with your help she will face it with faith and courage." Reagan died in 2004.

Never make [dementia] a secret. There
should be no shame. Why feel ashamed of
having a complex brain disease? People are
afraid to talk about it.
—WENDY MITCHELL

Sunday Times best-selling author, Wendy Mitchell, was diagnosed with young onset dementia at the age of 58. Wendy, who was a manager for 20 years until 2015, recalls: "I was coming out of my office one day and I didn't know who I was or who all the people around me were. It was only when she began meeting other people with dementia that her eyes were opened to the idea of being involved in research. She signed up to join Dementia Research and over time was invited to take part in a wide range of interesting studies. The results showed that the antibiotic did not significantly delay the progression of cognitive decline and functional impairment in people with Alzheimer's disease. Wendy Mitchell wrote her memoir after being diagnosed with Alzheimer's. That memoir, called *Somebody I Used to Know,* was published in 2018. Mitchell also blogs about her daily life with dementia.

> *In a funny way, Alzheimer's is perfect for celebrities. They greet people without being expected to know who those people are. They have brief, happy chats about nothing in particular. And then they move on, before anyone figures out that for people with Alzheimer's the small talk just gets smaller and smaller. The painful truth is that the woman who's greeting them so warmly has no idea what day of the week it is. She has no idea what year it is, either.*
>
> —DAN GASBY

Dan wrote about his famous wife, restaurateur, magazine publisher, celebrity chef, and nationally known lifestyle maven B. Smith, who struggled with memory loss in her 60's. His book, *Before I Forget,* is a look into the life they had and what it transformed into as her disease progresses.

What is Being Done?

I F YOU ARE INTERESTED in learning more about what the United States is planning, a good place to start is The National Plan, signed into law by President Obama in January 2011. It was the first nationally recognized plan the United States has ever had to address Alzheimer's. The goals are aggressive, and far reaching. Time will tell which goals are achieved, but a place to start was an achievement, and long overdue.

In the United States, attention to Alzheimer's disease took on heightened interest with passage of the National Alzheimer's Project Act (NAPA). Signed into law by President Obama in January 2011, the Act calls for an aggressive and coordinated national plan to accelerate research on Alzheimer's disease and related dementias, and to provide better clinical care and services for people living with dementia and their families.

Efforts under the National Plan are guided by an Advisory Council on Alzheimer's Research, Care, and Services, consisting of some of the Nation's foremost experts, convened by the Secretary of the U.S. Department of Health and Human Services. With the Advisory Council's guidance and public input, the first National Plan to Address Alzheimer's Disease was created in 2012.

The Plan establishes five ambitious goals to both prevent future cases of Alzheimer's disease and to better meet the needs of the millions of American families currently facing this disease:

- Prevent and effectively treat Alzheimer's disease by 2025
- Optimize care quality and efficiency
- Expand supports for people with Alzheimer's disease and their families
- Enhance public awareness and engagement
- Track progress and drive improvement

The National Institute of Health, NIH leads the research effort on the first goal, targeted at preventing and treating the disease. It is also where the largest amount of funding comes from. Updated annually, the research component of the National Plan is a collaborative, evolving framework. It outlines the basic, translational, and clinical research needed to understand and conquer Alzheimer's disease and related dementias. In support of the research goals of the National Plan, NIH embarked on an ambitious strategic planning process that engaged key stakeholders and resulted in the development of implementation milestones and success criteria.

In a recent TED Talk given by Samuel Cohen, he said, "It may surprise you that, put simply, Alzheimer's is one of the biggest medical and social challenges of our generation. But we've done relatively little to address it. Today, of the top 10 causes of death worldwide, Alzheimer's is the only one we cannot prevent, cure or even slow down. We understand less about the science of Alzheimer's than other diseases because we've invested less time and money into researching it." I could not agree more about the lack of attention this disease has received.

Who is Doing the Work?

It may be because I live primarily in Massachusetts that I am so aware of the good work that is being done in this field, and why I am so optimistic that a "cure," however that looks, will be found. Indeed, Massachusetts is the home of Harvard University, and global information analytics giant Elsevier, announced in 2019 that the United States is the world's top producer of Alzheimer's research, with Harvard leading the way. Incidentally, China is second, but with about half of the total output. In the report, they noted a trend they see that there is "increasing emphasis on topics like sleep, exercise, and keeping the brain active" according to then senior vice-president of Analytics for Elsevier, Maria De Kleijn-Lloyd.

US National Institutes of Health (NIH)

The biggest single funder for Alzheimer's research is the US National Institutes of Health (NIH), which is the primary agency of the United States government responsible for biomedical and public health research. It was founded in the late 1880s and is now part of the United States Department of Health and Human Services. The majority of NIH facilities are located in Bethesda, Maryland, and other nearby suburbs of the Washington metropolitan area, with other primary facilities in the Research Triangle Park in North Carolina and smaller satellite facilities located around the United States. The NIH conducts its own scientific research through the NIH Intramural Research Program (IRP) and provides major biomedical research funding to non-NIH research facilities through its Extramural Research Program.

As of 2013, the IRP had 1,200 principal investigators and more than 4,000 postdoctoral fellows in basic, translational, and clinical research, being the largest biomedical research institution in the world, while, as of 2003, the extramural arm provided 28 percent of biomedical research funding spent annually in the U.S., or about $26.4 billion.

The NIH comprises 27 separate institutes and centers of different biomedical disciplines and is responsible for many scientific accomplishments, including the discovery of fluoride to prevent tooth decay, the use of lithium to manage bipolar disorder, and the creation of vaccines against hepatitis,

Haemophilus influenzae (HIB), and human papilloma-virus (HPV).

Alzheimer's Disease Research Center at Mayo Clinic

The Alzheimer's Disease Research Center at Mayo Clinic promotes research and education about healthy brain aging, mild cognitive impairment, Alzheimer's disease, Lewy body dementia, frontotemporal dementia, and other related dementia disorders.

Alzheimer Disease International

ADI is the international federation of Alzheimer and dementia associations around the world, working in an official capacity with the World Health Organization. Their vision is risk reduction, timely diagnosis, care, and inclusion today, and cure tomorrow. They believe that tackling dementia requires efforts at global, regional, and local levels, and so we advocate at multilateral, bilateral and regional levels.

They work by empowering Alzheimer and dementia associations to advocate for dementia as a national priority, to raise awareness and to offer care and support for people with dementia and their care partners. Globally, they strive to focus attention on dementia, maintain it as a global health priority, campaign for better policy from governments and encourage investment and innovation in dementia research. Their work to empower Alzheimer and dementia associations includes our Alzheimer University, a series of practical workshops aimed at building and strengthening capacity in advocacy and policy, alongside care and support for people living with dementia, their care givers and family.

Following the adoption of World Health Organization's Global action plan on the public health response to dementia in 2017, ADI is working with our members to ensure that all countries in the world implement and fund dementia action plans, monitor their effectiveness, raise much needed awareness and help tackle stigma and is supported by their members and partners globally. ADI is the publisher of the World Alzheimer Report, the main creator globally of socioeconomic content on the condition, and provides commentary and information on developments in research, science, treatment, care, and innovation.

The Alzheimer's Association

The world's largest nonprofit funder of Alzheimer's research is the Alzheimer's Association, which is currently investing over $250 million in 750 active best-of-field projects in 39 countries. The Alzheimer's Association was founded by Jerome H. Stone with the help of several family members in Chicago, Illinois, and incorporated on April 10, 1980, as the Alzheimer's Disease and Related Disorders Association, Inc. It is a non-profit American volunteer health organization which focuses on care, support, and research for Alzheimer's disease.

The organization has chapters and communities across the nation, with its national office located in Chicago and the public policy office in Washington, D.C. Its mission is "to eliminate Alzheimer's disease through the advancement of research; to provide and enhance care and support for all affected; and to reduce the risk of dementia through the promotion of brain health."

American Brain Foundation

The American Brain Foundation was founded to bring researchers and donors together to cure brain diseases and disorders. Their mission statement: "For almost 30 years, we have funded research across a broad spectrum of brain and nervous system diseases and disorders in the pursuit of improved treatments, prevention, and cures. We focus on the full spectrum of brain diseases and disorders because we believe that when we cure one disease, we will cure many."

Cure Alzheimer's Fund

The vision for Cure Alzheimer's Fund was set by their founders. Frustrated with the slow pace of research about the disease, they applied their experience in venture capital and corporate startups to build an organization specifically designed to accelerate research, make bold bets, and eradicate the disease. Their mission statement is, "The organization's unwavering focus on finding a cure is made possible by our Board of Directors which finances our overhead expenses so that 100 percent of all donations go to support our research."

Alzheimer's Foundation of America

The mission of the Alzheimer's Foundation of America (AFA) is to provide support, services and education to individuals, families and caregivers affected by Alzheimer's disease and related dementias nationwide, and fund research for better treatment and a cure.

Fisher Center for Alzheimer's Research Foundation

The Fisher Center for Alzheimer's Research Foundation is an American nonprofit organization that supports research into the causes and treatment of Alzheimer's disease. The organization's mission is to "understand the causes of Alzheimer's disease, improve the care of people living with it, and find a cure."

> *The emotional center of the brain, the amygdala,*
> *never dies. Your mother may forget your name,*
> *but her "heart" understands who you are to her.*

—DR. PAUL RAIA

Advocacy and Informational Resources

I have compiled a wide variety of resources that may be of interest to friends, families, and caregivers of those diagnosed with Alzheimer's and of course to those who have themselves received this diagnosis and have a deep need to seek out information, and hope. It consists of recommended books to read, movies to watch, organizations to reach out to for help, and advocacy and research organizations to donate to. Additionally, I offer an overview of who is doing the desperately needed research on this foe. Please be so kind as to pass this book along to someone who has need of it if your family's journey is over.

Alzheimer's Association
225 N Michigan Ave
Chicago, IL 60611
24/7 Helpline 1-800-272-3900
www.alz.org

Alzheimer's Disease Education and Referral Center
(ADEAR)
800-438-4380
www.nia.nih.gov/alzheimers

Alzheimer's Foundation of America
322 Eighth Avenue, 7th Floor
New York, NY 10001
Helpline 1-866-232-8484
www.alzfdn.org

Alzheimer's Research Forum
www.alzforum.org

Cure Alzheimer's Fund
34 Washington St., Suite 310
Wellesley Hills, MA 02481
www.curealz.org

Family Caregiver Alliance
235 Montgomery Street, Suite 950
San Francisco, CA 94104
800-445-8106
www.caregiver.org

Lewy Body Dementia Association
912 Killian Hill Rd. SW
Lilburn, GA 30047
LBD Caregiver #: 800-539-9767
National Offices: 404-935-6444
www.lbda.org

MedicAlert Foundation
5226 Pirrone Court
Salida, CA 95368
800-432-5378
www.medicalert.org

UsAgainstAlzheimer's
P.O. Box 34565
Washington, DC 20043
www.usagainstalzheimers.org

UK Alzheimer's Society
www.alzheimersresearchuk.org

Alzheimer's and Dementia Help (UK)
www.alz.org.uk

Recommended Books on Family Caregiving

Activities to do with Your Parent who has Alzheimer's Dementia by Judith Levy North

User-friendly activities that will help maintain your parents' self-care skills, mobility, and socialization.

Alzheimer's Action Plan: The Expert's Guide to the Best Diagnosis and Treatment for Memory Problems by P. Murali Doraiswamy

Provides insights from a social worker and Alzheimer's disease expert on the diagnosis, best tests and medical treatment, coping, behaviors, clinical trials, informed consent, and more.

Alzheimer's Advisor: A Caregiver's Guide to Dealing with the Tough Legal and Practical Issues by James Vaughn

Covers legal implications, estate planning, advance directives, guardianship, legal liability, cost of care, caring for caregivers, and more.

Alzheimer's / Dementia Interactive Activity Books for Patients and Caregivers by Matthew Schneider and Deborah Drapac

Designed for memory-impaired adults and communication with people living with Alzheimer's, Parkinson's, stroke, brain injury, or related dementias, this eight book set provides sensory and cognitive stimulation for reminisce, recall, and sharing stories.

Alzheimer's Disease Sourcebook: Basic Consumer Health Information About Alzheimer Disease, Other Dementias, and Related Disorders by Karin Bellenir

A compendium of basic consumer health information about Alzheimer's disease and other dementias.

Alzheimer's Disease and Dementia: What Everyone Needs to Know by Steven Sabat

Providing an accessible primer on understanding what touches so many lives, this book contributes what is urgently missing from public knowledge: unsparing investigation of their causes and manifestations, and focus on the remaining strengths of the people diagnosed.

Alzheimer's Early Stages: First Steps for Family, Friends, and Caregivers by Dan Kuhn Almeda

In its 3rd edition, covers three key areas of the disease: medical aspects, day-to-day care, and care for the caregiver.

Better Living with Dementia: Implications for Individuals, Families, Communities, and Societies by Laura Gitlin and Nancy Hodgson

Practical applications for dementia care authored by experienced clinicians with information not covered in other resources.

Caregivers Guide to Dementia: Using Activities and Other Strategies To Prevent, Reduce, and Manage Behavioral Symptoms by Laura Gitlin and Catherine Verrier

This book thoroughly examines the strategies most helpful for preventing and managing behavioral symptoms such as agitation, depression, sleep disturbances and more.

Caregiver's Path to Compassionate Decision Making: Making Choices For Those Who Can't by Vicki Kind

Includes four adaptable tools and techniques for decision making for Alzheimer's, stroke, dementia, brain injury, mental illness and developmental delay.

Coping with Behavior Change in Dementia: A Family Caregivers' Guide by Beth Spencer and Laurie White Ann Arbor

The newest edition of the long-time standard *Understanding Difficult Behaviors* by Spencer, White, and Robinson. This version covers potentially difficult behaviors such as: bathing, dressing, eating, bathroom care, wandering or exercise, paranoia and delusions, and sleep and sundowning.

A Creative Toolkit for Communication in Dementia Care by Karrie Marshall

Tested through first-hand experience, the toolkit provides creative enterprises for communication and relating to the person with dementia by covering a wide range of activities.

Dignified Life: The Best Friends Approach to Alzheimer's Care by Virginia Bell and David Troxel

Based on the Best Friends model of care, the book focuses on creative and effective communication and meaningful activities.

Forget Me Not by Debra Kostiw

Drawing from the latest developments in Alzheimer's care, provides concise strategies to care for those with neurodegeneration.

The Everything Alzheimer's Book: Reliable, Accessible Information for Patients and Their Families by Carolyn Dean, M.D.

Authoritative information on the disease and its symptoms, treatments, and effective management.

Navigating Alzheimer's: 12 Truths About Caring For Your Loved One by Mary K. Doyle

This slim book is packed with snippets of real-life situations and solutions that have worked for the author.

Navigating the Alzheimer's Journey: A Compass For Caregiving by Carol Bowlby Sifton

Contains chapters on the disease, communication, management, behaviors, environment, capitalizing on remaining abilities, getting help, care planning and planning for the future.

Learning to Speak Alzheimer's by Joanne Koenig Coste

One of the first guides to changing the way care was delivered to people with dementia, and therefore a profoundly influential book. It teaches the now well understood "habilitation" approach.

Matters of the Mind and the Heart: Meeting the Challenges of Alzheimer's Care by Beverly L. Moore, RN

This slim book is a great first book to read as you begin to be a caregiver for someone with Alzheimer's.

Mayo Clinic on Alzheimer's and Other Dementias by Jonathan Graff-Radford, M.D., and Angela M. Lunde, M.A.

Are there ways you can lower your risk of dementia? Can it be prevented? Can you live well with dementia, if so, how? This book provides answers to these important questions and more.

The Mindful Caregiver by Nancy Kriseman

Helps caregivers identify unrealistic expectations, learn to set limits and more effectively cope with guilt and worry which can fuel caregiver stress.

Pocket Guide for the Alzheimer's Caregiver by Daniel C. Potts and Ellen Woodward Potts

Provides useful practical information for the newly diagnosed.

The 6 Steps to Managing Alzheimer's Disease and Dementia by Andrew E. Budsman, MD, and Maureen K. O'Connor, PsyD.

Comprehensive yet written in an easy-to-read style, this book features clinical vignettes and character-based stories that provide real-life examples of how to successfully manage Alzheimer's disease and dementia.

The 36-Hour Day by Nancy Mace and Peter Rabins

In its fifth edition, this comprehensive guide to the care of those in all stages of Alzheimer's disease combines practical advice and specific examples and covers the medical, legal, financial, and emotional aspects of caring.

Stages of Senior Care: Your Step-By-Step Guide to Making the Best Decisions by Paul Hogan

Provides chapters on all aspects of senior care and decision making.

How to Survive Caregiving: A Daughter's Experience by Cheryl Woodson West

A comprehensive and candid guide to the experience of care giving for everyone and especially those with an African American interest.

Recommended Books of Personal Stories

Before I Forget: Love, Hope, Help and Acceptance in Our Fight Against Alzheimer's by B. Smith, Dan Gasby and Michael Shnayerson

Restaurateur, magazine publisher, celebrity chef, and nationally known lifestyle maven B. Smith is struggling at 66 with a tag she never expected to add to that string: Alzheimer's patient. At its heart, *Before I Forget* is a love story illuminating a love of family, life, and hope.

Dementia Activist by Helga Rohra

In this book, single German mother Helga Rohra recounts her many experiences as an activist and advocate for people with dementia. She herself has a diagnosis of Lewy Body dementia.

Everything Left to Remember by Steph Jagger

This book is about the author's post-diagnosis journeys with her mother through several national parks, exploring life, the Rockies, memory's power, and relationships. Please enjoy her comments and consider reading her book.

Memory's Last Breath by Gerda Saunders

"My book is for this: to add my personal story to the body of science about dementia already accumulated by the lifetime of efforts of neuroscientists, neuropsychologists, other medical researchers and healthcare workers." At age 61, University of Utah professor Gerda Saunders was diagnosed with dementia. She resigned from her position and began to keep a journal that she called "Field Notes on My Dementia." This book is a mix of excerpts from this journal and fascinating accounts from her life which never stopped being adventurous.

On Pluto: Inside the Mind of Alzheimer's by Greg O'Brien with foreword by Lisa Genova

This book was written by Greg O'Brien, a fellow south shore resident, shortly after he was diagnosed with Alzheimer's. The places he visits, the restaurants, the locals, the doctors he consults are all familiar to me, so it was both interesting and deeply sad to follow another intelligent, lively person through the journey where I know how it ends. But he is so truly himself and original that it was so worth the read, and I think you will agree.

Slow Dancing with a Stranger: Lost and Found in the Age of Alzheimer's by Meryl Comer

Emmy-award winning broadcast journalist and leading Alzheimer's advocate Meryl Comer's *Slow Dancing with a Stranger* is a profoundly personal, unflinching account of her husband's battle with Alzheimer's disease that serves as a much-needed wake-up call to better understand and address a progressive and deadly affliction. With harrowing honesty, she brings readers face to face with this devastating condition and its effects on its victims and those who care for them.

Somebody I Used to Know: Wendy Mitchell

At 58 years old, Wendy Mitchell, from York, UK, received a diagnosis of Young Onset Dementia.

This book is largely autobiographical, documenting Wendy's life before and after a diagnosis of dementia. The writing is often poetic yet easy to read, and the messages are clear and poignant.

Still Alice by Lisa Genova

This extraordinary work of fiction, a New York Times bestseller, reads like a memoir, and is deeply, heartbreakingly realistic. The author uses her own experiences, having her character who lives in Boston and has a home on the Cape like the author, to make the story come alive with believable details. You will not forget it after you read it and will want others to read it, before they see the utterly wonderful movie.

Travelers to an Unimagined Land by Dasha Kiper

This book is told from a very unusual perspective that caregivers will appreciate. It explains exactly why a person with dementia may be doing things that the caregiver finds bewildering, especially at the early stages. The contrast between the healthy brain and the brain being taken over by Alzheimer's makes this a fascinating read.

This Room is Yours by Dr. Michael Stein

An unflinching look at a physician dealing directly with the effects of Alzheimer's on his mother, and the journey of finding an assisted living community for her. Weaving through the book is the important issue of coming to terms with their mother-son relationship.

The Forgetting: Alzheimer's: Portrait of an Epidemic by David Shenk

"I conceived of a book that might on the one hand, catalogue the horrors of Alzheimer's, and on the other, relay the hopeful story of the race to cure the disease. Instead, [I] realized that the story of Alzheimer's is in some ways exactly the opposite of my original premise: it is a condition specific to humans that, like nothing else, acquaints us with life's richness by ever so gradually drawing down the curtains."

Losing My Mind: An Intimate Look at Life with Alzheimer's by Thomas DeBaggio

This memoir begins with a 57-year-old man being tested for Early Onset Alzheimer's, and the story chronicles the journey of the author, who is the man being tested, as he gradually loses his memory. Moving and unusual.

We Are Not Ourselves by Matthew Thomas and Amanda Lang

This is an epic multigenerational portrait of the Irish American Leary family 'whose ambitions are tempered by a case of early onset Alzheimer's. This book took years to write, and the masterly result is well worth the read.

What the Hell Happened to my Brain? by Kate Swaffer

Kate was just 49 years old when she was diagnosed with a form of younger onset dementia. In this book, she offers an all-too-rare first-hand insight into that experience, sounding a clarion call for change in how we ensure a better quality of life for people with dementia. A must read for people with dementia and their families as well as for professionals and carers.

Recommended Films

Age Old Friends (1989)

Hume Cronyn achieves another great performance as John Cooper, who chose to live in a retirement home instead of with his daughter (played by real-life daughter Tandy Cronyn), as a symbol of maintaining his independence. He befriends Michael (Vincent Gardenia), who starts showing signs of dementia. When John's daughter extends an offer to live with her again, John must decide between leaving the rigid structure of the retirement home and staying to help his friend cope with his disease.

Alive Inside: A Story of Music and Memory (2014)

This American documentary directed and produced by Michael Rossata-Bennett premiered at the Sundance Film Festival and was an audience favorite. It explores the stories of patients and their experiences with music therapy.

Away From Her (2007)

In "Away from Her," Julie Christie was Oscar-nominated for Best Actress for her portrayal of Fiona, a woman with Alzheimer's who voluntarily enters a care facility to avoid being a burden on Grant, her husband of 50 years. After a 30-day separation (recommended by the facility), Grant visits Fiona and finds that her memory of him has deteriorated and that she's developed a close friendship with another man in the facility. Grant must draw upon the pure love and respect he has for Fiona to choose what will ensure his wife's happiness in the face of the disease. Christie won a Golden Globe Award for Best Actress in a Motion Picture (Drama) for her performance in this movie.

Determined: Fighting Alzheimer's (2022)

"Determined: Fighting Alzheimer's" premiered on the PBS series NOVA Wednesday, April 6, 2022. Filmed over five years, this is an independent documentary portraying the stories of three women and their decision to participate in Alzheimer's disease research. The film features research participants and scientists at the Wisconsin Registry for Alzheimer's and is an intimate look at three women, Barb, Karen, and Sigrid, who participate in the WRAP research study and return every two to three years to undergo a multidisciplinary oral cognitive test. This battery of questions looks for problems with their memory that could be a signal of their worst fear—the onset of Alzheimer's disease.

The Father (2020)

In "The Father," Anthony Hopkins plays a man with dementia who begins to challenge himself and his loved ones as he exhibits his raw emotions about his disease, his daughter moving away, and life in general. Hopkins received an Oscar for Best Performance. The film, which was inspired by director and co-writer Florian Zeller's personal experience with a grandmother who had Alzheimer's, won Oscars for Best Adapted Screenplay and during the 2021 British Academy Film Awards the movie won for both Best Performance and Best Adapted Screenplay.

First Cousins Once Removed (2013)

This deeply moving and thought-provoking documentary by acclaimed filmmaker Alan Berliner chronicles his mother's first cousin, the well-known poet Professor Edwin Honig, on his journey into the depths of Alzheimer's.

Iris: A Memoir of Iris Murdoch (2001)

Based on the book "Elegy for Iris" by John Bayley, this movie tells the true story of English novelist Iris Murdoch's descent into Alzheimer's disease and the unconditional love of Bayley, her partner of 40 years. Jim Broadbent won an Academy Award and a Golden Globe for Best Supporting Actor for his portrayal of Bayley in his later years. Judi Dench and Kate Winslet received both Academy Award and Golden Globe nominations for Best Actress and Best Supporting Actress, respectively, for their portrayal of Murdoch in her older and younger years.

The Iron Lady (2011)

The film is based in the present day and features flashbacks to Lady Thatcher's early life, her rise to power and the defining events of her premiership and downfall. From the opening scene, where a confused and befuddled Lady Thatcher wanders into a corner shop to buy a pint of milk, the film begins to show Lady Thatcher battling with Dementia.

It Snows all the Time (2023)

Screenwriter and actor Erich Hover said about his new film: "Both of my grandmothers had Alzheimer's disease. In 2010, my dad received his own diagnosis at age 58, after having a PET scan. I truly didn't realize that this could happen to someone so young. My misconceptions about the disease, paired with my dad being in the prime of his life—working full-time, traveling, reading, working out daily—made his diagnosis hit differently."

Memory (2022)

Memory is an American action thriller film directed by Martin Campbell from a screenplay by Dario Scardapane. It is based on the novel De Zaak Alzheimer by Jef Geeraerts and is a remake of the novel's previous adaptation, the Belgian film The

Alzheimer Case. The film stars Liam Neeson as an aging hitman with early onset dementia who must go on the run after declining a contract on a young girl.

The Notebook (2004)

Based on Nicholas Sparks' best-selling novel of the same name, "The Notebook," this beloved movie features James Garner as Noah, the loving husband of Allie (Gena Rowlands), who is in a nursing home due to Alzheimer's disease. Noah attempts to rekindle her memories of their long history by reading to her from his notebook. Ryan Gosling and Rachel McAdams play the couple in their younger years.

Poetry (2010)

This is a South Korean drama written and directed by Lee Chang-dong. It tells the story of a suburban woman in her 60s who begins to develop an interest in poetry while struggling with Alzheimer's disease and her irresponsible grandson. Yoon Jeong-hee stars in the leading role, which was her first role in a film since 1994. The film was selected for the main competition at the 2010 Cannes Film Festival, where it won the Best Screenplay Award.

The Savages (2007)

Laura Linney and Philip Seymour Hoffman play siblings in this tragic yet comedic film about adult children caring for a parent with dementia. Laura Linney was Oscar-nominated for Best Actress, and Tamara Jenkins was Oscar-nominated for Best Original Screenplay. With a rare combination of humility, dignity, and humor, Philip Seymour Hoffman was Golden Globe-nominated for Best Actor in a Motion Picture for his touching performance as the neurotic professor who begrudgingly unites with his sister for the sake of their father.

A Song for Martin (2001)

Sven Wollter and Viveka Seldahl play married couple Martin and Barbara in this Swedish movie with English subtitles. Martin is a conductor and composer while Barbara is a world class violinist. They meet and marry in middle-age, but soon after, they find out that Martin has Alzheimer's disease. This touching story is considered by many to be one of the most realistic depictions of caregiving on film.

Still Alice (2014)

In this movie, based on Lisa Genova's 2007 best-selling book of the same name, Julianne Moore stars as Alice Howland, a professor diagnosed with early-onset Alzheimer's disease. Her husband is played by Alec Baldwin, and her children are played by Kristen Stewart, Kate Bosworth, and Hunter Parrish. This is based on a work of fiction and has a hopeful undertone.

Still Mine (2012)

Still Mine follows the story of Craig Morrison (James Cromwell), an elderly farmer trying to build a new home for him and his wife, Irene (Geneviève Bujold). The unexpected hurdles that are preventing him from going through with his plan and the unexpected issues that surface with Irene's progressing dementia demand that Craig compromise on certain things and to let go of others.

Supernova (2021)

Supernova is a fictional account inspired by the experiences of the writer and director, Harry Macqueen, while volunteering with people with dementia. Macqueen wrote and directed the tender story of Sam (Colin Firth) and Tusker (Stanley Tucci), partners for two decades who we meet on a road trip across England. In the film, Stanley Tucci portrays the lead character, Tusker, who has been diagnosed with dementia. It chronicles how he and his partner deal with the journey of being patient and caregiver. The film was awarded Best Feature at the European Film Festival.

What They Had (2018)

This American drama was written and directed by Elizabeth Chomko and stars Hilary Swank, Michael Shannon, Robert Forster, Blythe Danner, Taissa Farmiga and Josh Lucas. The film had its premiere at the Sundance Film Festival. The movie dramatizes Ruth, who suffers from Alzheimer's wandering out in a blizzard on Christmas Eve. Daughter, Bridget Ertz travels back to her hometown to help her brother, Nicky, convince their father to put Ruth in a nursing home and face the end of their lifelong love affair.

Acknowledgments

The only rule you need to know when interacting with someone with Alzheimer's is the golden rule. First educate yourself about what they are going through, then treat them as you would want to be treated in the same circumstances.

—SHARON RICARDI

I AM HAPPY THAT I COULD bring this collection of wisdom and resources to those that need it. I am only able to write about this subject, which has become so near and dear to my heart over these many years, due to my many teachers. I would like to publicly say thank you to some of my very first teachers; I received training to become a certified dementia practitioner many years ago from the wonderful Dr. Paul Raia of the Massachusetts Alzheimer's Association, and the late Joanne Koenig Coste who later wrote her groundbreaking book, *Speaking Alzheimer's*, about her husband's journey. They were wonderful, caring teachers. I would be remiss not to mention my former colleague, the inimitable Marilyn Stasonis, who had us all "stepping into their reality" and picturing the brain as a big onion. And this, from a friend who wishes to remain anonymous:

> *I describe the process of getting a diagnosis as death by a thousand cuts. One test leads to another test, and then another and another. You know you didn't ace them, and that feeling multiplies with each test you undergo. But you keep taking them, still keep hoping it will end with a conversation with your doctor that starts with "I'm happy to tell you that you've been needlessly worried." But that did not happen. I knew in my heart it wouldn't. Eventually the only thing left to say was that "it's probably Alzheimer's.*

—AN ANONYMOUS FRIEND

Thank you of course to my wonderful children and family and supporters who encouraged and aided me in this process. Special thanks to Lee Lyman, my love, for your support all along the way; and the many others who believed in the project and helped push me to finish: Jim, Wendy, Greg, Holly, Andra, Richard, and Karen.

Be well,
Sharon

About the Author

Sharon Ricardi has over 30 years of experience in the field of health care and senior care, specializing in Alzheimer's disease. As the president of Northbridge Advisory Services, she and her staff travel to clients nationally and advise them on operational issues, especially those focusing on memory care. She has given many talks and been a featured panelist and speaker at such national trade conferences as NIC, Senior Living 100, Senior Living Innovation Forum, Argentum, and more.